Respiratory Medicine

Series Editors

Sharon I.S. Rounds
Alpert Medical School of Brown University
Providence, RI, USA

Anne Dixon
University of Vermont, Larner College of Medicine
Burlington, VT, USA

Lynn M. Schnapp
University of Wisconsin - Madison
Madison, WI, USA

More information about this series at http://www.springer.com/series/7665

Dee W. Ford • Shawn R. Valenta

Editors

Telemedicine

Overview and Application in Pulmonary,
Critical Care, and Sleep Medicine

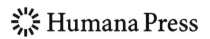

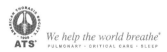

We help the world breathe®
PULMONARY · CRITICAL CARE · SLEEP

Editors
Dee W. Ford
Medical University of South Carolina
Charleston, SC
USA

Shawn R. Valenta
Medical University of South Carolina
Johns Island, SC
USA

ISSN 2197-7372   ISSN 2197-7380   (electronic)
Respiratory Medicine
ISBN 978-3-030-64049-1   ISBN 978-3-030-64050-7   (eBook)
https://doi.org/10.1007/978-3-030-64050-7

This Humana imprint is published by the registered company Springer Nature Switzerland AG
The registered company address is: Gewerbestrasse 11, 6330 Cham, Switzerland

Preface

When we embarked on editing a telehealth book, we could not have envisioned the rapid uptake in telehealth that would occur associated with the COVID-19 global pandemic. Our original vision was to provide an introductory overview of themes relevant to virtually all telehealth programs along with a detailed examination of telehealth in pulmonary, critical care, and sleep medicine. We have termed the first part of this book a telehealth "primer." The objective of the primer is not to provide a comprehensive manual on telehealth, but is to give readers a valuable overview of topics that need to be considered, addressed, and adapted to the reader's local context. Primer topics include an overview of the history of telehealth, regulatory/legal issues, financial considerations, historical challenges to telehealth service development and implementation, technology considerations, people factors in telehealth, and how telehealth can drive quality in healthcare. The second section provides an evidence-based review of telehealth services in select pulmonary/sleep medicine topics including pediatric asthma, home-based chronic obstructive pulmonary disease management, and sleep disordered breathing. This is followed by a detailed chapter on telemergency including examples of triage tools for telemergency programs. Finally, the book concludes with a chapter on tele-ICU, arguably the area with the most robust evidence base. We hope readers find this a useful introduction to this important topic and an area of indisputable growth in healthcare.

Charleston, SC, USA   Dee W. Ford
Johns Island, SC, USA   Shawn R. Valenta

Contents

Editors

Dee W. Ford, MD, MSCR Medical University of South Carolina, Charleston, SC, USA

Shawn R. Valenta, MHA Medical University of South Carolina, Johns Island, SC, USA

Contributors

Annie Lintzenich Andrews, MD, MSCR Department of Pediatrics, Medical University of South Carolina, Charleston, SC, USA

Bryan T. Arkwright, BS, MHA Cromford Health, Charlotte, NC, USA

School of Law, Wake Forest University, Winston-Salem, NC, USA

Partners in Digital Health/Telehealth and Medicine Today Journal, New York, NY, USA

Danielle K. Block, BS UMMC Center for Telehealth, University of Mississippi Medical Center, Jackson, MS, USA

Elizabeth A. Brown, PhD, MPA Department of Health Professions, Medical University of South Carolina, Charleston, SC, USA

Michael Caputo, MS Department of Information Technology, Marist College, Poughkeepsie, NY, USA

Gerard J. Criner, MD, FACP, FCCP Department of Thoracic Medicine and Surgery, Lewis Katz School of Medicine at Temple University, Temple University Hospital, Philadelphia, PA, USA

Ragan DuBose-Morris, EdS, PhD Academic Affairs Faculty, Center for Telehealth, Medical University of South Carolina, Charleston, SC, USA

Kyle Faget, JD Telemedicine and Digital Health Industry Team, Foley & Lardner, LLP, Boston, MA, USA

Alexis E. Frehse, MHA Phillips Gilmore Oncology Communications, Inc., Philadelphia, PA, USA

Meghan Glanville, MHA MUSC Center for Telehealth, Medical University of South Carolina, Charleston, SC, USA

Tina Sweeney Gustin, DNP, CNS, RN Center for Telehealth Innovation, Education and Research, College of Health Sciences, Department of Nursing, Old Dominion University, Virginia Beach, VA, USA

Jillian B. Harvey, MPH, PhD Department of Healthcare Leadership and Management, Medical University of South Carolina, Charleston, SC, USA

Michael Haschker, AA (Electronic Engineering) Telehealth Technologies, Department of Information Solutions, Medical University of South Carolina, Charleston, SC, USA

Daniel M. Hynes, MD Department of Pulmonary, Critical Care, Allergy, and Sleep Medicine, Medical University of South Carolina, Charleston, SC, USA

Jessica Joseph, JD Telemedicine and Digital Health Industry Team, Foley & Lardner, LLP, Boston, MA, USA

Akram Khan, MD (MBBS) Department of Pulmonary Critical Care, Oregon Health & Sciences University, Portland, OR, USA

Kathryn L. King, MD, MHS Department of Pediatrics, Medical University of South Carolina, Charleston, SC, USA

Isabelle Kopec, MD Department of Critical Care, Advanced ICU Care, Creve Coeur, MO, USA

Nathaniel M. Lacktman, JD Telemedicine and Digital Health Industry Team, Foley & Lardner, LLP, Tampa, FL, USA

Chitra Lal, MD, FCCP, FAASM, FACP, ATSF Department of Pulmonary, Critical Care, Allergy and Sleep Medicine, Medical University of South Carolina, Charleston, SC, USA

Morgan E. Light, MS, BA, BS, BSN Department of Surgical Intensive Care, Wake Forest Baptist Medical Center, Winston-Salem, NC, USA

Claire A. MacGeorge, MD, MSCR Department of Pediatrics, Medical University of South Carolina, Charleston, SC, USA

Nandita R. Nadig, MD, MSCR Department of Medicine, Medical University of South Carolina, Charleston, SC, USA

Monica L. Nash, MHA Department of eHealth, SCP Health, Mobile, AL, USA

Gustavo Adolfo Fernandez Romero, MD Department of Thoracis Medicine and Surgery, Lewis Katz School of Medicine at Temple University, Temple University Hospital, Philadelphia, PA, USA

Emily Sederstrom, MHA Department of Strategic Planning, OU Medicine, Oklahoma City, OK, USA

Alexandra Shalom, JD Telemedicine and Digital Health Industry Team, Foley & Lardner, LLP, Boston, MA, USA

Sarah A. Sterling, MD Department of Emergency Medicine, University of Mississippi Medical Center, Jackson, MS, USA

Richard L. Summers, MD Department of Emergency Medicine, University of Mississippi Medical Center, Jackson, MS, USA

Kathy Hsu Wibberly, PhD Karen S. Rheuban Center for Telehealth, Mid-Atlantic Telehealth Resource Center, University of Virginia School of Medicine, Charlottesville, VA, USA

Part I
Primer on Telemedicine Program Development

Chapter 1
Overview and History of Telehealth

Alexis E. Frehse

Brief History of Telehealth

1950s

By most accounts, it appears that the 1950s was the decade when contemporary telehealth began in the United States and Canada. In fact, 1950 was the year that telemedicine was first mentioned in medical literature [1]. In addition to being included in a medical publication, live, two-way telehealth visits were occurring at the University of Nebraska by the end of the decade.

In the year 1959, visits were occurring on campus between clinical instructors and their medical students [1]. The telehealth practice in Nebraska began with neurological exams and then expanded to include group therapy consultations. This demonstrates that even in its earliest stages, telehealth was being utilized to not only expand access to care, but also to expand education efforts. Toward the end of the decade, Canadian radiologists began to experiment with telehealth utilizing fluoroscopy images (i.e., an X-ray movie) to diagnose patients [1].

1960s

In the 1960s, the first instances of asynchronous or store-and-forward telehealth were recorded through the transmission of X-rays and electrocardiograms [1]. In these early instances, telehealth was used to diagnose patients at sea while the provider remained on shore. This decade also experienced a boom in live, synchronous

A. E. Frehse (✉)
Phillips Gilmore Oncology Communications, Inc., Philadelphia, PA, USA
e-mail: afrehse@phillipsgilmore.com

© Springer Nature Switzerland AG 2021
D. W. Ford, S. R. Valenta (eds.), *Telemedicine*, Respiratory Medicine,
https://doi.org/10.1007/978-3-030-64050-7_1

telehealth in not only rural areas, but also urban areas with a need for immediate medical care. One system that did notable work in this field was Massachusetts General Hospital (MGH). In 1963, MGH established (through telecommunications) a medical outpost at Logan Airport in Boston that was staffed by nurses to treat patients in emergency situations. Five years later, efforts were expanded and the service evolved into telehealth that included the use of a stethoscope during the live, interactive consultation [1].

But MGH was not the only organization to expand telehealth efforts; in 1964, the Nebraska Psychiatric Institute received a grant from the US National Institute for Mental Health (NMH) that allowed the institute to experiment with a pilot program in which they connected to Norfolk State Hospital. The program provided education and consultations from specialists at the Nebraska Psychiatric Institute to general practitioners at Norfolk State Hospital [2]. Once again, illustrating how the educational aspect of telehealth is continuously and consistently integrated with the clinical aspect. Throughout the evolution of telehealth, the clinical and educational components continue to grow and progress simultaneously.

1970s

Telehealth efforts expanded exponentially in the 1970s mainly due to the involvement of federal agencies including the National Aeronautics and Space Administration (NASA) and the US Department of Health, Education, and Welfare (currently the Department of Health and Human Services, DHHS). In 1972, both agencies launched their own separate programs [2].

NASA's program was titled Space Technology Applied to Rural Papago Advanced Health Care (STARPAHC), and it was an initiative that connected healthcare providers to patients in remote areas with little or no access to healthcare. Patient sites, defined as originating or presenting sites, were located in paramedic vans and connected with medical providers at hospitals in Tucson and Phoenix, Arizona [2]. Members of the Papago Indian Reservation as well as astronauts benefitted from this NASA iniative, which endured for nearly 20 years [1].

DHHS's program involved seven different projects that included research as well as clinical care. The project partners included the following:

- Illinois Mental Health Institutes in Chicago
- Ohio's Case Western Reserve University in Cleveland
- Massachusetts' Cambridge Hospital, Illinois
- Bethany/Garfield Medical Center in Chicago
- Minnesota's Lakeview Clinic in Waconia
- Dartmouth Medical School's INTERACT in Hanover, NH
- Mount Sinai School of Medicine in New York City [2]

The success of the partnerships led to two additional telehealth projects in the states of Florida and Massachusetts that were funded by the US National Science Foundation (NSF) [2]. Not wanting to be outdone by their neighbors to the South, the Canadian Space Program partnered with Memorial University of Newfoundland to pilot their own telehealth initiative utilizing the Hermes satellite, which was shared with the United States [2].

1980s

In the 1980s, telehealth began to expand on a global scale with the implementation of programs in Australia, Armenia, and Russia [2]. In Australia, telehealth programs were developed based on a need for providing care to patients in rural areas.

In the country of Armenia, the need arose due to the occurrence of a natural disaster. An earthquake, occurred in 1989, and led to the utilization of telehealth between the United States and Yerevan, Armenia. The visits were set up for one-way, asynchronous communication, and allowed for consultations from four major medical systems in the United States facilitated through a Joint Working Group on Space Biology between the United States and Armenia. This eventually led to an international partnership between the United States and Russia, when the telehealth services offered to Armenia were then extended to Russia through the Space Bridge Program [2].

In the United States, the Department of Defense (DOD) partnered with the Public Health Service to enhance Tele-Radiology efforts for civilians and military personnel [1].

While the 1970s witnessed the rapid development and expansion of telehealth programs, the early to mid-1980s witnessed a significant slowdown. Many attribute this to the growing cost of the equipment as well as the complexity of the associated technology. However, by the end of the decade, things began to accelerate yet again as technology improved and equipment became more economical [1].

1990s

The 1990s brought a technology boom with the invention of the Internet or the World Wide Web (as it was commonly known then). In this decade, the American Telemedicine Association (ATA) was established, and the DHHS created the Office for the Advancement of Telehealth (OAT). Telehealth expanded so quickly that it was no longer possible to keep an inventory or database of all the emerging programs [3]. In addition to the expansion, this decade saw more diverse telehealth programs emerging as well as the creation of the first affiliations of separate academic medical institutions.

One notable example of an affiliation involving telehealth is Telequest, which was a Tele-Radiology program established by five academic medical centers:

- Bowman Gray
- Brigham and Women's Hospital
- Emory University
- University of California at San Francisco
- University of Pennsylvania [1]

Examples of other diverse telehealth programs that evolved in this decade include the following:

- Direct-to-consumer telehealth services
- Telehealth services into prisons
- Tele-psychiatry
- Telehealth services into skilled nursing facilities

In fact, the term "electronic housecall" was coined in the 1990s to identify this new mode of telehealth delivery [1].

The idea of utilizing telehealth to care for the prison population was gaining popularity due to substantial cost-savings and alleviation of safety concerns. In 1995, it was estimated that in the state of North Carolina it cost more than $700 to transport a prisoner to the hospital to receive care. By participating in telehealth programs, states such as North Carolina, Colorado, and Texas were able to reduce these costs considerably [1]. In addition to providing cost-savings, the use of telehealth programs to treat the prison population greatly decreased the number of individuals who could potentially escape and cause harm to others. This second benefit alleviated safety concerns previously held when seeking medical care for a member of the prison population.

While the concept of tele-psychiatry was not a new concept, it did experience growth and advancement through a program in Oregon called Rural Options for Development and Education Opportunities (RODEO NET). This program received a $700,000 grant from the Office of Rural Health Policy (ORHP) in 1991 and used it to expand and sustain its program. The program was so successful that it became self-sustaining and no longer depends on grant funding [1].

Finally, the idea of post-surgical follow-up through telehealth in a skilled nursing facility setting developed into a program through a partnership between Stanford University Medical Center and Lytton Gardens Health Care Center. The program began with a focus on post-transplant patients and expanded to reconstructive surgery patients and then vascular surgery patients. The partnership was mutually beneficial. Stanford University Medical Center decreased the length of stay for the patient, and Lytton Gardens Health Care Center experienced the benefits of improved reimbursement from treating more complex patients [1]. As a result, appropriate and efficient care was delivered at both facilities.

2000s

In the new millennium, government and regulatory agencies begin to catch up to the rapid expansion of telehealth. In this decade, state governments and medical boards begin to develop and establish their own telehealth policies [4].

In 2005, Kentucky became the first state to establish its own network, the Kentucky Telehealth Network. Kentucky's original parity law required payers to reimburse telehealth services at the same rate as in-person services as long as the provider was in-network and affiliated with the Kentucky Telehealth Network [5].

In 2006, six regional Telehealth Resource Centers (TRCs) were established by the Health Resources Services Administration (HRSA) to assist with the development and implementation of telehealth programs throughout the United States. The TRCs were funded by grants through the DHHS of about $300,000 per year and remain an invaluable resource for organizations seeking to learn about telehealth broadly as well as regional. The centers also assist with questions regarding any state-specific issues for their respective regions [6].

The passing of the American Recovery and Reinvestment Act of 2009 (ARRA) continued the advancement and expansion of telehealth through its focus on the need for increasing the utilization of electronic health records (EHR) and/or electronic medical records (EMR) [7]. Through the ARRA, $17 billion was allocated to update health technology systems and several more billions were allocated to scientific research [7]. An impactful component of the ARRA was the Health Information Technology for Economic and Clinical Health Act (HITECH), which further prompted the shift to electronic medical records allowing the exchange of medical information in a more efficient and secure manner [8].

2010s and the Future

The current decade continues the theme of regulation from the previous decade. The Affordable Care Act (ACA), passed in 2010, continues the apportionment of federal dollars to telehealth programs and services. There is also an increased focus on the triple aim:

- Improving population health
- Enhancing the patient care experience
- Reducing per capita cost

Telehealth is viewed as an important component to many strategies seeking to achieve the triple aim. In response to the growing demand for telehealth services, six additional telehealth resource centers were established through grants of nearly $400,000 per year in 2014, bringing the total number of federally funded regional TRCs to 12 in addition to two national telehealth resource centers, the Center for Connected Health Policy and the National Telehealth Technology Assessment Resource Center [6].

In 2017, the Health Resources and Services Administration (HRSA) awards the designation of national Telehealth Centers of Excellence to the Medical University of South Carolina and the University of Mississippi Medical Center [9]. This award is the first of its kind and allows for the continuation of research and development of telehealth technology and best practices. Telehealth technologies continue to develop, and the telehealth market is projected to grow to almost $2 billion [10].

This decade also witnessed a surge in the development and utilization of mobile applications or as they are more commonly referred to as apps. In 2016, over a quarter of a million apps related to health and wellness were available for download [11]. The popularity of healthcare apps can be attributed to the popularity of wearable smart devices, such as Fitbits and Apple watches. The majority of mHealth apps can be classified into one of the seven buckets listed as follows [11]:

- Chronic care management apps—Medical apps
- Healthcare and fitness apps
- Women's health apps
- Medication management apps
- Personal health record apps
- Patient education apps

The apps that fall into these various buckets can help with a wide array of healthcare-related issues, such as tracking one's steps for the day, to helping manage a chronic condition such as diabetes, or to monitoring a patient's recovery after a major surgery.

As a component of assisting with patient treatment and care, mHealth apps can allow patients to have easy and immediate access to their medical record. Patients also have the ability to get in touch with their provider to ask questions or request a medication refill anytime and anywhere. In some instances, patients can even use an app to launch a live, two-way telehealth consult or submit a healthcare questionnaire with corresponding photos [11]. Researchers expect to see the mHealth app market reach $111.8 billion by the year 2025 [11]. This is largely driven by consumer demand as applications continue to make things easier and more convenient.

As technology becomes increasingly integrated into everyday life, it has been assumed that telehealth will become a social norm, completely integrated with other elements of health. Similarly to how talking on the phone has evolved into video conferencing or how various platforms and applications are used for common activities, such as requesting transportation or shopping, healthcare will likely follow suit. Ultimately, when healthcare is needed, options for delivery of that care will be considered and the need for in-person evaluation will be one of a variety of technology enabled choices.

In the coming decades, as healthcare strives toward achieving the triple aim, the need to ensure access to the same effective and efficient care regardless of patient location will grow increasingly important.

What Is and Is Not Telehealth?

As telehealth continues to gain popularity and become more commonplace the question of what is and is not telehealth continues to arise. Is telemedicine the same as telehealth? Are the two terms interchangeable? If not, what are the key differences between the two?

In 2014, the federal government of the United States sought to answer these questions. As a result, a special task force was convened to "identify and evaluate the definitions of telemedicine/telehealth across the U.S. Government to provide a better understanding of what each agency or department means when it uses these terms" [12].

The work group brought together over 100 participants from the federal departments of Health and Human Services, Defense, Justice, Labor, Transportation, Veterans Affairs, Agriculture, Commerce, as well as several independent agencies [9]. The aim of this section is to clearly define what is and is not telehealth.

Telemedicine is defined by the Health Resources and Services Administration (HRSA) as:

> the use of electronic information and telecommunications technologies to support and promote long-distance clinical health care, patient and professional health-related education, public health and health administration. Technologies include videoconferencing, the internet, store-and-forward imaging, streaming media, and terrestrial and wireless communications. [13]

The definition above can apply to both telemedicine and telehealth and the ATA goes as far as to state that the two terms can be used interchangeably [12]. Similarly, a World Health Organization (WHO) report in 2010 noted that for the purposes of the report the two terms "are synonymous and used interchangeably" [12].

However, this has not always been the case. Historically, telemedicine has been viewed as consultation and diagnosis between a provider and a patient or a consultation between two providers (i.e., second opinion). Some even go as far to say that telemedicine is specifically the interaction between the patient and a physician, and telehealth encompasses all other types of providers (i.e., physician assistants, nurse practitioners, and registered dieticians).

As a part of the initiative, the federal work group was tasked with soliciting definitions for the following terms: telemedicine; telehealth; telemonitoring; telepresence, store-and-forward; and mhealth from all federal groups [14]. Telehealth was the term that received the most responses, and it was discovered that six definitions of the term were used across seven different offices in the Department of Health and Human Services alone [14].

Upon discovering this, the work group decided to focus on the similarities and differences of the terms used in each definition [14]. The results showed that most definitions included healthcare services and education [14].

Telehealth has been historically viewed as the educational component and is defined by the federal telehealth group as "a broader concept than telemedicine and addresses the use of information technologies not only for delivering medical care remotely, but also for delivering preventive health and other public health interventions remotely" [14]. This educational/public health branch includes training for healthcare professionals such as emergency medical technicians, nutrition and fitness classes taught by a registered dietician, or even long-distance learning opportunities between several healthcare professionals in both domestic and international settings.

More recently, the idea of wellness has gained momentum as there has been an influx of healthcare apps that track steps, caloric intake, and heart rate. Since these apps are rarely vetted or reviewed by physicians, they more often than not fall into the more general telehealth category.

Another aspect in the debate of what is and is not telehealth includes the platform or specific technology that is used as the channel of communication. It is critical that the technology selected for use is secure and HIPPA-compliant. Some providers are quick to recommend that a patient text a picture or take it upon themselves to utilize FaceTime to observe, diagnose, and provide follow-up care to patients. These forms of technology are neither considered secure nor HIPPA-compliant and can create significant compliance risks. They also present issues when attempting to bill for professional fees and other forms of telehealth reimbursement that may be available through third-party payers.

Conversely, the use of appropriate technology does not necessarily mean that the communication and/or interaction is telehealth. For example, the use of HIPPA-compliant technology to connect to grand rounds or a departmental meeting is not and should not be considered telehealth.

To conclude, the terms "telemedicine" and "telehealth" are generally synonymous just as the use of the medical and healthcare fields are considered interchangeable. It is important to note the historical differences between the two terms and understand that the currently suggested term "telehealth" can encompass all facets of health and wellness. As the shift toward preventive health continues to occur, it is crucial that health include not only medical care, but also wellness.

Modes of Telehealth Delivery

When identifying the four key modes of telehealth delivery, it is important to remember that telehealth is not a practice in-and-of itself, but it is a tool to improve the efficiency and/or effectiveness of care. It is not a new type of healthcare, but simply a different way to deliver the same or higher quality care.

While many automatically think of telehealth as a live, two-way video conference with one's provider, there are actually four main modes that encompass the methods that a patient can receive care via telehealth. Broadly considered, telehealth interactions are categorized with regard to timing and with respect to the

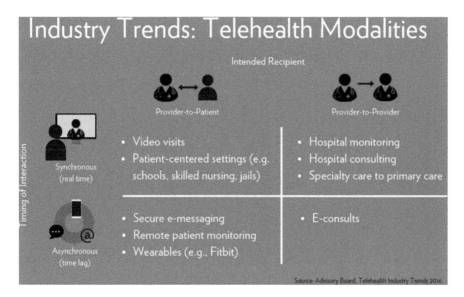

Fig. 1.1 Telehealth interactions by timing and intended recipient

intended recipient. With regard to timing, telehealth interactions may occur either synchronously or asynchronously. With regard to intended recipients, these may be between patients and providers or provider-to-provider. See Fig. 1.1 for examples, several of which are explained below [13].

Synchronous (Live, Two-Way), Videoconferencing

Synchronous videoconferencing is traditional telehealth and what comes to mind when many hear the phrase "telehealth." In this situation, the patient is located at the originating or presenting site and the provider is located at the distant site.

The mode of delivery can include a provider-to-provider connection or a patient-to-provider connection. In some situations, a tele-presenter (oftentimes a medical assistant or nurse) can work with the remote provider to conduct a physical exam and help to evaluate the patient through the use of telehealth peripheral devices. These devices include items such as a stethoscope and/or otoscope.

Asynchronous and/or Store-and-Forward

The asynchronous method has gained popularity in recent years and involves asynchronous communication between the provider and the patient or between two providers. It differs from synchronous because it is not live, does not include video communication, and does not promote immediate interaction.

This type of telehealth can be used in a variety of ways for a variety of specialties. Some organizations utilize asynchronous telehealth methods to evaluate images, such as, tele-radiology or tele-EEG. Other organizations utilize it as a solution to evaluate and treat non-acute conditions, such as upper respiratory tract symptoms or minor skin rashes. Treatment can be streamlined by the completion of a questionnaire and when applicable, the submission of an image by the patient. This particular use-case, sometimes termed tele-urgent or virtual urgent care, has gained substantial traction in recent years and represents one of the fasted growing segments in telehealth [15]. Finally, an important type of telehealth collaboration between two providers, termed "e-consults" or more recently by CMS "internet interprofessional consultations" serves to garner a second opinion in a more efficient manner. Due to the potential for this type of telehealth to reduce unnecessary sub-specialty referrals and/or decrease wait times for needed specialty referrals, this is a venue closed health systems, such as, the Veterans Administration have long embraced with positive results. The availability of new professional fee billing codes under CMS should prompt organizations with relatively deep sub-specialty resources to consider how to strategically develop and deploy services in this telehealth category.

Remote Patient Monitoring

Remote patient monitoring involves a provider at the distant site monitoring and acting upon patient data from the originating or presenting site. Such data might include hemodynamic parameters, blood glucose levels, and other provider or patient-reported measures. Additionally, the provider can assist the staff at the originating site and provide direction in critical and urgent situations. This mode of telehealth delivery is most commonly used in two distinct clinical contexts—chronic disease management and tele-ICU services. The latter is extensively reviewed in Chapter 12.

Mobile Health or mHealth

Mobile health involves the use of mobile devices, such as smart phones and tablets, and it is the method that has gained the most popularity in recent years. In fact, a report in 2014 noted that 84 percent of patients aged 18–34 preferred a consultation through a mobile device [16].

The same report notes that there are over 100,000 mHealth apps on the market and that the use of these apps has grown at a rate of 87 percent when compared to the general app industry [16]. The use of the mHealth telehealth delivery mode can be extremely helpful for monitoring chronic conditions such as diabetes and/or obesity. It can also be extremely effective in serving as a conduit to facilitate communication between the provider and the patient in a secure and safe manner.

Mobile health or mHealth can also be used as a tool to monitor patients at home after major medical events such as surgery. There is also growing interest in the role of apps to more successfully manage specific patient populations and decrease emergency department visits and admissions. For example, a patient undergoing heart surgery may be asked to download an app as a part of the recovery process. By collecting and analyzing weight, blood pressure, and blood oxygen levels, through the app, providers can allow patients to recover in the comfort of their home and also maintain a watchful eye during the recovery process. The access to the data and established parameters allows the provider to better manage the patient and adjust medication and care accordingly. Once again achieving the overall goal of telehealth by delivering care in a more efficient and effective manner.

Conclusion

As telehealth continues to grow and evolve, providers and healthcare systems must envision how telehealth can be utilized to improve quality of care from a multi-stakeholder perspective, which includes patients, providers, payers, and health systems. As healthcare increasingly shifts toward value-based care, telehealth will play a key role in improving population health. Furthermore, the combination of technologic advancements and patient demand will drive ongoing innovation.

References

1. Field MJ. Telehealth: a guide to assessing telecommunications in health care. Washington, D.C.: National Academy Press; 1997.
2. Allan R. A brief history of telemedicine [Internet]. Electronic Design. 2012 [cited 2018Jun12]. Available from: http://www.electronicdesign.com/components/brief-history-telemedicine.
3. Maheu MM, Alen A, Whitten P. E-health, telehealth and telemedicine: a guide to start-up and success. San Francisco: Jossey-Bass; 2001.
4. Stateline. Can telemedicine be the future of health care? [Internet]. The Huffington Post. TheHuffingtonPost.com; 2015. Available from: https://www.huffingtonpost.com/entry/can-telemedicine-be-the-future-of-health-care_us_562f9186e4b06317990f6673.
5. Restrepo K. The case against telemedicine parity laws [Internet]. John Locke Foundation. John Locke Foundation; 2018 [cited 2018 Jun 12]. Available from: https://www.johnlocke.org/research/telemedicine/.
6. The Federally Funded Telehealth Resource Centers [Internet]. www.cchpca.org. Center for Connected Health Policy; 2014. Available from: http://www.cchpca.org/sites/default/files/resources/PERSPECTIVESARTICLECCHP-FederallyFundedTRCs2014.pdf.
7. Amadeo K. What did ARRA really do? [Internet]. The Balance. The Balance; [cited 2018 Jun 12]. Available from: https://www.thebalance.com/arra-details-3306299.
8. HHS Office of the Secretary, Office for Civil Rights, OCR. HITECH act enforcement interim final rule [Internet]. HHS.gov. HHS.gov; 2017. Available from: https://www.hhs.gov/hipaa/for-professionals/special-topics/hitech-act-enforcement-interim-final-rule/index.html.

9. UMMC, MUSC Recognized as Telehealth Centers of Excellence [Internet]. Healthcare Informatics Magazine. Available from: https://www.healthcare-informatics.com/news-item/telehealth/ummc-musc-recognized-telehealth-centers-excellence.
10. Vogel LH. Telemedicine. In: Who knew?: inside the complexity of American Health Care. Boca Raton: CRC Press; 2019. p. 51.
11. Hassan Mansoor [Internet]. CustomerThink. 2018. Available from: https://customerthink.com/how-mobile-health-apps-for-patients-change-the-mhealth-trends/.
12. mHealthIntelligence. Is there a difference between telemedicine and telehealth? [Internet]. mHealthIntelligence. 2016. Available from: https://mhealthintelligence.com/features/is-there-a-difference-between-telemedicine-and-telehealth.
13. Telemedicine and Telehealth [Internet]. HealthIT.gov. Available from: https://www.healthit.gov/topic/health-it-initiatives/telemedicine-and-telehealth.
14. Doarn CR, Pruitt S, Jacobs J, Harris Y, Bott DM, Riley W, et al. Federal Efforts to define and advance telehealth—a work in Progress. Telemed J E Health. 2014;20(5):409–18.
15. Gordon AS, Adamson WC, DeVries AR. Virtual visits for acute, nonurgent care: a claims analysis of episode-level utilization. J Med Internet Res. 2017;19(2):e35. https://doi.org/10.2196/jmir.6783. PMID: 28213342; PMCID: PMC5336603. https://www.healthaffairs.org/doi/abs/10.1377/hlthaff.2017.1087?journalCode=hlthaff.
16. The Rise of mHealth: 10 Trends [Internet]. Becker's Hospital Review. Available from: https://www.beckershospitalreview.com/healthcare-information-technology/the-rise-of-mhealth-10-trends.html.

Chapter 2
Telehealth Legal and Regulatory Issues

Kyle Faget, Nathaniel M. Lacktman, Jessica Joseph, and Alexandra Shalom

Abbreviations

ABMS	American Board of Medical Specialties
ACGME	Accreditation Council for Graduate Medical Education
AKS	Anti-Kickback Statute
AOA	American Osteopathic Association
AOABOS	American Osteopathic Association Bureau of Osteopathic Specialists
CAHs	Critical Access Hospitals
CMIA	Confidentiality of Medical Information Act
CMPs	Civil Monetary Penalties
CMS	Centers for Medicare & Medicaid Services
COMLEX-USA	Comprehensive Osteopathic Medical Licensing Examination of the United States
CSA	Controlled Substances Act
DEA	Drug Enforcement Agency
FCC	Federal Communications Commission
FDA	The Food and Drug Administration
FTC	Federal Trade Commission
HIPAA	The Health Insurance Portability and Accountability Act of 1996
IMLC	Interstate Medical Licensure Compact
OIG	Office of Inspector General
PC	Professional Corporations

K. Faget (✉) · J. Joseph · A. Shalom
Telemedicine and Digital Health Industry Team, Foley & Lardner, LLP, Boston, MA, USA
e-mail: kfaget@foley.com

N. M. Lacktman
Telemedicine and Digital Health Industry Team, Foley & Lardner, LLP, Tampa, FL, USA

© Springer Nature Switzerland AG 2021
D. W. Ford, S. R. Valenta (eds.), *Telemedicine*, Respiratory Medicine,
https://doi.org/10.1007/978-3-030-64050-7_2

PHI   Protected Health Information
Stark Laws   Ethics in Patient Referrals Acts of 1989
TCPA   Telephone Consumer Protection Act
USMLE   United States Medical Licensing Exam

Telehealth and Physician Licensure

General Physician Requirements

All physicians are required to comply with the state licensure requirements of the state(s) where they practice medicine. However, additional considerations apply when a physician provides telehealth services to patients in another state. In that case, the question generally becomes whether the physician is licensed in the state where the patient is located.

The requirements for telehealth licensure vary from state to state, and differing state medical practice standards can add additional obstacles for physicians looking to practice across state lines. Most states require physicians to be fully licensed in the state where a patient is located before providing care to that patient, but not all states explicitly address the provision of telehealth services in relevant licensing statutes. Where states do not specifically address telehealth in their licensing statutes, it should be assumed that a full license is needed to provide telehealth services to patients located in those states. Other states, such as Alabama and Texas, allow physicians to obtain special purpose licenses in order to practice telehealth in their state [1, 2].

Exceptions to Physician State Licensure

Some states have certain exceptions to licensing requirements in specific circumstances. One such example is the bordering state exception, which some states employ to allow physicians from bordering states to practice across state lines. For example, Virginia provides license reciprocity for physicians providing telehealth services to patients in Virginia if the physician is licensed in a bordering state, which includes Maryland, Washington D.C., North Carolina, Tennessee, Kentucky, and West Virginia [3].

Other exceptions include the peer-to-peer consultation exemption, where out-of-state physicians who are consulting with a physician in a given state need not be licensed in that state. In these circumstances, the out-of-state physician typically must be licensed in the state where he or she is located, and the in-state physician must be licensed in the state where he or she and the patient are located. The in-state physician is held responsible for maintaining the physician-patient relationship, while the out-of-state physician's services are only for secondary consultation purposes. Though the in-state physician always maintains primary responsibility for patient care, some states with peer-to-peer consultation exceptions allow the out-of-state physician to have direct contact with the patient, provided that this contact is infrequent or is at the direction of the in-state physician. For example, in Minnesota, an out-of-state physician providing telehealth services is exempt from licensure in Minnesota if the physician is licensed in another state and (1) provides services less than once a month or to less than ten patients per year or (2) provides services in consultation with a Minnesota-licensed physician who "retains ultimate authority over the diagnosis and care of the patient" [4].

The scope of the peer-to-peer consultation exemption varies greatly between states. In Connecticut, a physician who provides only "irregular" consultations is exempt from state licensure requirements, though "irregular" is not defined, while in Iowa, state law specifically requires that a physician "practices in Iowa for a period not greater than 10 consecutive days and not more than 20 total days in any calendar year" to be exempt [5, 6]. Michigan only permits exceptions for physicians providing consultations in "an exceptional circumstance," and Alabama specifies that an exception only applies when the physician does not receive compensation for the consultation [7, 8]. Thus, it is vital for any physician to consult the specific rules of the state in which they wish to provide telehealth services.

Interstate Medical Licensure Compact

The Interstate Medical Licensure Compact (the "IMLC") offers a new expedited route to licensure for certain physicians who seek to practice in multiple states. Currently, 29 different states, the District of Columbia, and Guam have signed on to the IMLC; under this agreement, eligible physicians can obtain licenses to practice medicine in those states within the IMLC [9]. The IMLC allows an eligible physician's application to be expedited by leveraging the existing information previously submitted by that physician in his or her state of principal license.

In order to be eligible for the IMLC route, a physician must (1) hold a full, unrestricted medical license in a member state, and either live, work, or conduct at least 25% of their practice of medicine there; (2) have graduated from an accredited medical school or an eligible international medical school; (3) successfully completed ACGME or AOA accredited graduate medical education; (4) passed each component of the USMLE, COMLEX-USA, or equivalent in no more than three attempts; (5) hold a current specialty certification or time-unlimited certification by an ABMS or AOABOS board; (6) have no history of disciplinary action toward his or her medical license; (7) have no criminal history; (8) have no history of controlled substance actions toward his or her medical license; and (9) not currently be under investigation. Physicians who are not eligible for the expedited process can still seek additional licenses in member states using the traditional state-by-state licensure process. As additional states enact the IMLC, the more coordinated the process of interstate medical licensure and practice will become.

Telehealth and State Physician Practice Standards Laws

Telehealth Modalities and Creating a Valid Doctor-Patient Relationship

Treating patients via telehealth necessarily includes use of various communication technologies to facilitate patient consultation, diagnosis, education, treatment, and general patient management. These treatment modalities include, but are not limited to, live audio-video communications, mobile health, store-and-forward, and remote patient monitoring, including wearable technologies. Interactive audio-video communication allows for real-time patient interaction and, in some instances, may serve as a substitute for an in-person visit. Mobile health enables physician practices to communicate with patients via cell phones and tablet personal computers, which can be extremely useful for communication of information such as public health announcements. Store-and forward involves the asynchronous transmission of a patient's recorded health history, for example, X-rays and photographs, to the treating physician. Remote patient monitoring involves the ongoing collection and transmission of patient-level data at one location to another where a health care provider can access and utilize the data for managing chronic conditions and making treatment decisions.

While in some cases, the treatment modality chosen may reflect the most efficient and cost-effective approach to patient management and treatment, in other cases the treatment modality selected may be influenced by factors such as a practitioner's ability to secure coverage for services. For example, under the Medicare conditions of payment for telehealth services and following satisfaction of the applicable geographic and scope of service restrictions, the applicable coverage rules outside the context of a public health emergency require communication between a patient and a practitioner to occur via a real-time interactive audio and video telecommunication system [10]. These conditions of payment, therefore, render treatment using audio-only, store and forward,[1] or mobile communication modalities ineligible for Medicare coverage as a telehealth service.

Informed Consent

Because telehealth is a relatively new approach to the delivery of health care, practitioners should consider use of an informed consent with patients, explaining in plain terms what telehealth is, the expected benefits, the potential risks, the limitations, and alternatives to receiving care via telehealth. While no federal law exists

---

[1] CMS does allow the use of asynchronous "store and forward" technology for delivering telehealth services when the originating site is a Federal telemedicine demonstration program in Alaska or Hawaii. *See* 42 CFR 410.78(d).

requiring health care providers to obtain informed consent for telehealth, states and payers often have specific requirements regarding telehealth informed consent. At the state level, consent requirements appear in statutes, administrative codes, and/or Medicaid policies. For example, under MaineCare Medicaid, a health care provider must obtain an informed consent signed by the member or his or her legally authorized representative in advance of providing any telehealth services [11]. Additionally, the informed consent must be retained as part of the member's medical record and provided to the member or the member's legally authorized representative upon request [11].

State-specific informed consent requirements can also vary according to the type of service being performed, the modality being utilized, and the requirements for documentation and retention. The Kentucky Board of Medical Licensure, for example, stipulates that a proper telehealth informed consent should include, among other things, information regarding identification of the patient, the physician's name and credentials, the types of transmissions permitted using telehealth technologies, agreements that a treating physician determine the appropriateness of use of telehealth for the condition being diagnosed or treated, and details on security measures taken to secure telehealth technologies being utilized, namely, encrypting data [12]. State informed consent requirements are evolving as telehealth becomes integral to mainstream medical practice. In California, telehealth informed consent requirements were revised by Assembly Bill No. 809, which permits consent to be obtained verbally or in writing so long as the consent is documented, and by abandoning the requirement that the health care provider who obtains the consent be at the originating site where the patient is physically located. Failure to comply with the California informed consent requirement constitutes unprofessional conduct.

Standard of Care

"Standard of care" is typically defined as the level and type of care a reasonably competent and skilled health care professional would deliver to a patient under similar circumstances. In addition to state medical boards holding providers accountable for meeting the standard of care, standard-of-care deviations form the basis for medical malpractice claims. Understanding how standard of care shifts and/or remains the same in the context of telehealth is critical for health care providers engaged in the practice of telehealth.

The level and type of care required in the traditional care context is largely determined by local customs, which may include local and/or federal practice standards. For telehealth, where the health care provider and patient do not share the same location, application of local custom can be challenging, but certain standards have emerged as nearly universal. With respect to telehealth, many states posit that "the standard of care is the same whether the patient is seen in-person, through telemedicine or other methods of electronically enabled health care" [13, 14].

Specific Disclosures and Record Sharing Requirements

Telehealth providers are subject to state laws relating to medical record documentation and retention requirements. In general, telehealth documentation retained in a patient's medical record must be as detailed as an in-person office visit. For example, the Texas Administrative Code states, "documentation in the patient's medical record for a telehealth medical service or a telehealth service must be the same as for a comparable in-person evaluation" [15]. In addition to the requirement that patient medical records include "copies of all relevant patient-related electronic communications, including relevant patient-physician e-mail, prescriptions, laboratory and test results, evaluations and consultations, records of past care and instructions," the Texas Administrative Code notes, "If possible telemedicine encounters that are recorded electronically should also be included in the medical record" [16]. Under the Iowa Administrative Code, the telehealth requirements for medical records are quite specific.

A licensee who uses telemedicine shall ensure that complete, accurate, and timely medical records are maintained for the patient when appropriate, including all patient-related electronic communications, records of past care, physician-patient communications, laboratory and test results, evaluations and consultations, prescriptions, and instructions obtained or produced in connection with the use of telemedicine technologies. The licensee shall note in the patient's record when telemedicine is used to provide diagnosis and treatment. The licensee shall ensure that the patient or another licensee designated by the patient has timely access to all information obtained during the telemedicine encounter. The licensee shall ensure that the patient receives, upon request, a summary of each telemedicine encounter in a timely manner [17].

The telehealth medical record documentation and retention requirements are, at a minimum, parallel to those of an in-person encounter. In some cases, they are more onerous because the practitioner may be expected to designate details regarding the use of telehealth and store electronic recordings.

Telehealth Prescribing

State Laws

All states allow prescribing via an authentic telehealth encounter in the context of a valid physician-patient relationship. What is required to form a valid physician-patient relationship varies from state to state, and impacts the ease with which telehealth may be utilized. With a certain number of caveats, most states do not require an in-person examination to establish a physician-patient relationship. Iowa-licensed physicians, for example, may establish a valid physician-patient relationship "through telemedicine, if the standard of care does not require an in-person encounter, and in accordance with evidence-based standards of practice and tele-medicine practice guidelines that address the clinical and technological aspects of telemedicine" [18]. It follows that Iowa allows remote prescribing of non-controlled substances without a prior in-person examination provided that, before administer-ing treatment or issuing prescriptions, an Iowa-licensed physician interviews the patient to collect the relevant medical history and performs a physical examination, when medically necessary, sufficient for the diagnosis and treatment of the patient [19].

Controlled Substances and the Federal Ryan Haight Act

Following the situation where a young man overdosed on painkillers purchased via the internet in 2001, Congress responded by signing into law the Ryan Haight Online Pharmacy Consumer Protection Act (21 U.S.C. § 802(54)) (the "Ryan Haight Act") in 2008. The Ryan Haight Act amended the federal Controlled Substances Act (21 U.S.C. § 802 *et seq.*) (the "CSA") by prohibiting the dispensing of controlled substances via the internet unless the prescriber previously conducted at least one in-person medical evaluation of the patient. Although exceptions were made to allow the use of telehealth during the Public Health Emergency related to COVID-19 [20] and under highly specific circumstances to prescribe controlled substances,[2] few allow for remote prescribing via modern applications of telehealth. While the Ryan Haight Act may have addressed rogue internet prescribing prac-tices, it also has had the effect of chilling legitimate telehealth practice. Rural com-munities who often have little to no access to psychiatric care, for example, would benefit from remote prescribing of controlled substances but for the existence of the Ryan Haight Act.

A number of states, including Indiana, Hawaii, and Florida, have begun to address the limitations that the Ryan Haight Act places on telehealth. For example, in 2017, Indiana expanded the list of drugs that may be prescribed by authorized prescribers via telehealth to include certain controlled substances while placing lim-its on prescribing practices with respect to opioids, abortion inducing drugs, and ophthalmic devices [21]. Physicians engaging in remote prescribing of controlled substances risk being subjected to an enforcement action by the Drug Enforcement

---

[2]The exceptions include the following: the patient is being treated by and physically located in a hospital or clinic registered under 303(f) of the CSA (21 U.S.C. 823(f)); the patient is being treated by and in the physical presence of a practitioner; the telehealth practitioner is an employee or con-tractor of the Indian Health Service or tribal organization; the telehealth encounter is being con-ducted during a medical emergency as declared by the Secretary of Health and Human Services or a Department of Veterans Affairs medical emergency; the telehealth practitioner has obtained a special registration from the U.S. Attorney General; or the telehealth encounter is being conducted under circumstances that the U.S. Attorney General and the Secretary of Health have, jointly and by regulation, determined [22].

Agency ("DEA"), the agency charged with enforcing the Ryan Haight Act, even if such prescribing is permissible under state law.

Following the White House's 2017 declaration that the opioid crisis is a national public health emergency, the Acting Health and Human Services Secretary made a declaration under Section 319 of the Public Health Service Act, which allowed an exception to the Ryan Haight Act that would allow health care providers to prescribe controlled substances using telehealth without first conducting an in-person visit. This declaration could have cleared the way for DEA to remove restrictions associated with remote prescribing of controlled substances for the treatment of opioid addiction, but DEA did not issue a concurring declaration. Nonetheless, efforts are underway to align federal law with current telehealth practice. Two recently released draft federal discussion bills, "Improving Access to Remote Behavioral Health Treatment Act," [23] which would permit remote prescribing of controlled substances in the context of community mental health centers and addiction treatment centers without an in-person exam and "Special Registration for Telemedicine Clarification Act," which calls upon the Attorney General to promulgate regulations allowing for remote prescribing of controlled substances without the inclusion of a required in-person exam, aim to alleviate some of the consequences of the Ryan Haight Act by providing greater access to telemedicine.

Privacy and Security

Health Insurance Portability and Accountability Act (HIPAA) and Telehealth

HIPAA regulates the use and disclosure of protected health information ("PHI") that is held by certain covered entities, including health insurers, health care providers who submit claims electronically, health care clearinghouses, and employer-sponsored health plans, as well as by their contractors (who are "business associates"). It also sets out specific administrative, physical, and technical security safeguards for electronic PHI. HIPAA applies to covered entities in the telehealth setting, just as it does for traditional in-person medical care. Providers must take the same care when storing electronic patient files, images, and audio/video tapes as they would with paper documents, and all patient data that is transferred electronically must be secured.

Telehealth providers should ensure that their telehealth operations are secure and that no PHI is accidentally exposed to third parties or is vulnerable to third-party access, errors, or outages, which could lead to the loss or alteration of clinical data. Because these types of incidents may be potential HIPAA violations, adequate encryption and other protections are vital to ensure compliance with HIPAA.

Exceptions to HIPAA

HIPAA does not apply if no PHI is being exchanged. Moreover, HIPAA does not apply to every entity that collects a patient's identifiable health-related data, but only to specified Covered Entities and their Business Associates. Many patients and providers use their mobile devices, such as smartphones or tablets, to communicate, share data, and even make diagnoses via mobile health applications. Developers of these applications frequently are *not* Covered Entities subject to HIPAA rules—they are not health insurers or health care clearinghouses, for example, and they also do not qualify as business associates of covered entities such that HIPAA would apply. The particular nature and function of each app affects whether HIPAA applies in a given context. A wearable health app used by a consumer would not necessarily be subject to HIPAA, while an app that assists a physician in following up with patients likely should be designed to comply with HIPAA.

However, even if HIPAA does not apply, telehealth providers must ensure that they comply with applicable state law, as an increasing number of states have their own privacy and security statutes, which can be broader than HIPAA. In California, for example, the Confidentiality of Medical Information Act ("CMIA") has its own standards for permissible uses and disclosure of medical information. While CMIA was previously limited to the same types of entities that were subject to HIPAA, it was later amended to expand its scope to cover mobile health application developers. Many other states have enacted similar laws, requiring certain entities to comply with specific privacy and security requirements even if they are not subject to HIPAA. As such, it is important for telehealth providers to ensure they are up to date on HIPAA and whether it applies to them, as well as the relevant laws in the states in which they practice.

E-Commerce, the Telephone Consumer Protection Act (TCPA), and Privacy Policies

Various federal agencies issue regulations and enforce laws that may apply to telehealth providers. For example, the Federal Trade Commission ("FTC") enforces the FTC Act, which prohibits deceptive and unfair trade practices in commerce. These include practices relating to privacy and data security, such as a provider's misleading claims about a mobile health app's safety or performance. The FTC has also issued a Health Breach Notification Rule, which requires certain businesses to provide notifications after breaches of personal health data. The Food and Drug Administration ("FDA") enforces the Food, Drug, and Cosmetic Act, which regulates the safety and effectiveness of medical devices, including some mobile health apps.

The Federal Communications Commission ("FCC") is responsible for overseeing both interstate and international communications, and thus regulates communication devices transmitting medical data.

The FCC also administers the Telephone Consumer Protection Act ("TCPA"), which was enacted to protect consumer privacy by restricting unsolicited contacts from automated telephone calls, fax machines, and automatic dialers. Businesses cannot call, text, or fax consumers to solicit business unless they have been given express consent to do so. However, the FCC has created some exceptions applicable to the health care industry. Providers may send artificial or prerecorded voice messages or text messages to land lines and cell phones, without any prior consent, if those messages are regarding certain important health care information. The exception covers messages relating to lab results, prescription notifications, appointments and exams, confirmations and reminders, and home health care instructions, among others.

These exceptions do have restrictions, however. For example, voice calls and text messages can only be sent to the telephone number provided by the patient and must not include any telemarketing, solicitation, advertising, accounting, billing, or financial content. Moreover, a health care provider may only initiate one message per day (up to three per week) and each message must be concise in length. These messages must also include an easy way for patients to opt out of messages. Providers must honor these opt-out requests immediately.

Given the various laws and regulations regarding data privacy and security that affect the telehealth industry, it is important that providers develop robust privacy policies to ensure that all sensitive data is adequately protected. Telehealth providers should inform patients what specific data is collected—particularly any PHI pursuant to HIPAA—as well as the purposes for which patient data is used. Privacy policies should also inform patients about whether any patient-provided data is shared with third parties and the circumstances in which this information may be disclosed. It is also wise to inform patients of the risks in using telehealth services, given that no communication mechanism can ever be completely secure, as well as how patients can report suspected or actual breaches of security to the telehealth provider.

Because of the number of state and federal laws impacting data privacy and security in commerce, and specifically in the health care context, it is essential that those in the telehealth industry stay up to date on the relevant laws affecting the areas in which they provide services.

Malpractice Insurance Coverage and Tort Liability in Telehealth

Malpractice Insurance Coverage

Physicians providing medical services through telehealth must be cognizant of the risk of malpractice suits. Telehealth practitioners may be sued for a variety of mistakes including a misdiagnosis or a medication error. As such, physicians should investigate whether their malpractice insurance covers the scope of their telehealth services. This is especially true for practitioners who are providing services to patients in states where they are not licensed. For example, Colorado requires that out-of-state physicians who provide telehealth services to in-state patients maintain the same amount of malpractice insurance as physicians licensed and located in Colorado. As such, a physician may need to obtain additional or extended malpractice insurance coverage based on state-specific requirements.

Tort Liability

Medical malpractice occurs when a health care practitioner harms a patient through a negligent act or omission. In the health care setting, there must be an established physician-patient relationship to prove that a doctor owed a duty to his or her patient. According to the American Medical Association's Code of Medical Ethics, "a patient-physician relationship exists when a physician serves a patient's medical needs" [24].

In addition to proving that a physician-patient relationship exists, a potential patient litigant must also demonstrate that the physician's medical services fell below the applicable standard of care. The applicable standard of care is constantly evolving and varies based on factors, including the services provided and state guidelines.

Some states have codified standards of care for telehealth. For example, Alabama, California, Florida, Kentucky, and North Carolina all view telehealth as a tool that aids in the practice of medicine rather than being the practice of medicine itself. These states apply the same standard of care for telehealth practitioners as for traditional in-person interactions [25–30]. These uniform standards of care apply to all aspects of the medical service, including patient verification, record keeping, and how and where to conduct a patient exam. Other states have only implemented specific standards for certain types of telehealth services such as prescriptive practices. Further, some states dictate the specific technological mechanisms that telehealth practitioners are required to use. In Idaho, practitioners must perform telehealth consults with audio-video communications if the practitioner has not previously performed an in-person examination [31].

Whenever new technology is introduced in the health care setting, it begs the question of whether the use and implementation of the technology will change the current standard of care. For example, an Emergency Medicine physician at rural hospital might satisfy the standard of care even if she fails to consult with a specialist to help diagnose and treat a stroke patient if there are no neurologists on staff. However, if the rural hospital gains access to remote neurologists through telehealth, that same physician may now fall below the standard of care if she fails to utilize this technology. As such, practitioners should stay current with evolving technology in their fields and local telehealth resources that change over time.

Hospital Credentialing of Telehealth Physicians

Overview

Hospitals are required by both the Centers for Medicare & Medicaid Services (CMS) Conditions of Participation and by the Joint Commission Standards to have a process for credentialing and privileging its physicians and practitioners. This requirement extends to practitioners who provide services through telehealth.

Prior to 2011, CMS required the same credentialing and privileging process for physicians and practitioners who were providing in-person services as for those who were providing virtual services. This was a poor allocation of resources because those who could benefit from telehealth services were deterred by the administrative process and associated costs. Small hospitals and Critical Access Hospitals ("CAHs") in need of specialty practitioner expertise were especially burdened by the cumbersome requirements. CMS realized that its uniform credentialing and privileging process was inhibiting the expansion of telehealth services. Therefore, CMS promulgated new regulation allowing for "credentialing by proxy." The new regulations, which are described below, give providers increased flexibility in hospital telehealth arrangements allowing for innovative patient-service delivery.

Credentialing by Proxy

In 2011, the Federal government promulgated the credentialing by proxy regulations to streamline the process for privileging and credentialing telehealth providers [32, 33]. Credentialing by proxy dramatically reduces the administrative burden on a hospital or a CAH that receives telehealth services ("Originating Site" hospital). If certain requirements are met, credentialing by proxy allows an Originating Site hospital to use the privileging and credentialing decisions from the hospital or entity ("Distant Site" hospital or entity) that is providing the services.

The Originating Site hospital must have a written agreement with the Distant Site hospital or entity that lays out the specific credentialing by proxy requirements:

1. The Distant Site hospital or entity's credentialing and privileging program meets or exceeds the traditional Medicare standards.
2. Each practitioner that provides telehealth services to the Originating Site hospital must be privileged at the Distant Site hospital or entity [34].
3. The Distant Site hospital or entity must provide the Originating Site hospital with the current list of the privileges for the practitioners providing telehealth services [34].
4. Each practitioner providing telehealth services is licensed to practice in the state where the Originating Site hospital is located [34].

5. The Originating Site hospital must periodically review the services the telehealth practitioners provide to its patients and allow the Distant Site hospital or entity to use this information in performance evaluations. These reports must include all adverse events or complaints for a telehealth practitioner's services that were provided at the Originating Site hospital [34].

6. Agreements with Distant Site entities must state that the Distant Site entity is a contractor of services for the Originating Site hospital and that it will furnish the contracted telehealth services in a way that allows the Originating Site hospital to comply with Medicare Conditions of Participation [34].

Ultimately, the Originating Site hospital retains authority over the privileging decisions its telehealth-based practitioners even when credentialing by proxy. As such, an Originating Site Hospital should have provisions about credentialing by proxy in its medical staff bylaws. In addition, an Originating Site hospital may want to create a separate classification for its telehealth providers that enumerates their responsibilities and rights.

Entities should remember that they always have the option to use the traditional credentialing and privileging process. Even if a hospital enters into a credentialing by proxy agreement with a Distant Site hospital or entity, the Originating Site hospital can opt out of the process for as many telehealth practitioners as it wants.

Other Notable Laws and Regulations Relevant to Telehealth

Corporate Practice of Medicine

Many states prohibit corporations from practicing medicine. The goal of the prohibition is to prevent laypersons (individuals not licensed to provide health care services) from interfering with a physician's medical judgment when making treatment decisions. Generally, the prohibition on the corporate practice of medicine prevents any entity that is owned by laypersons from delivering medical services and/or employing physicians. As such, medical personnel must be employed by physician-owned professional corporations ("PC"). Sometimes these prohibitions extend further and restrict who can employ other health care practitioners such as nurses, psychologists, or therapists.

The definition of practicing medicine and the exceptions to the prohibition vary dramatically by state. For example, many states exempt hospitals from these rules and allow them to employ physicians. Further, a layperson is allowed to own a medical group in Florida so long as the group completes a site survey and obtains a Health Care Clinic License. Other states do not have prohibitions on the corporate practice of medicine, and, in contrast, some states are known to strictly enforce their prohibitions on the corporate practice of medicine. California, New Jersey,

New York, Tennessee, and Texas all have a particularly strong history of enforcement. As such, telehealth practices that deliver services to multiple states should be cognizant of the variations in the rules on the corporate practice of medicine.

Federal Fraud and Abuse Laws: Stark, Anti-Kickback Statute, Civil Monetary Penalties

The Federal government has enacted a variety of laws to prevent fraud and abuse in the health care space. These include the Stark Laws, Anti-Kickback Statute (AKS), and the Civil Monetary Penalties (CMPs). There are many aspects of these laws that they remain unclear when applied in the telehealth setting. As such, practitioners should evaluate the risks of their proposed telehealth arrangement under each law.

Stark Laws and Telehealth

The Ethics in Patient Referrals Acts of 1989, more commonly known as the "Stark Laws" prohibit physicians from referring Medicare and Medicare beneficiaries to entities providing reimbursable designated health services with which the physician or an immediate family member have a financial relationship [35]. These referrals may still take place if an exception is met. Although the Stark Laws are narrow, they use a strict liability standard that does not require intent.

In the telehealth context, Stark may be implicated if a hospital and a physician have financial ties and the physician subsequently makes referrals for certain medical services at the hospital. However, a number of Stark exceptions may protect a hospital and physician that enter such an arrangement. Examples of such exceptions include bona fide employment, incidental medical staffing benefits such as pagers and internet access, and renting equipment. In addition, there are exceptions for electronic prescribing items and electronic health record items. Further, the community-wide health information systems exception allows physicians to refer Medicare patients to entities even if the physician received information from technology equipment or services that allow him or her to access and share electronic health records.

Anti-Kickback Statutes

The AKS makes it a crime to knowingly offer or receive remunerations for the purpose of inducing referrals for items or services reimbursable by a Federal health care program such as Medicare and Medicaid [36]. Although the AKS prohibition is broader than the Stark Law, there are safe harbors that protect certain arrangements from implicating the AKS statute. For example, there are safe harbors surrounding the use of electronic prescribing items and services and electronic health records [37].

Civil Monetary Penalties

The Civil Monetary Penalties (CMPs) is a broad law that authorizes the Secretary of Health and Human Services to impose civil money penalties and program exclusion for various forms of fraud and abuse involving a Federal health care program [38]. For example, CMPs may be assessed if false claims for payment are presented or are caused to be presented for payment by the Federal government. The beneficiary inducement provision of the CMP prohibits offering or transferring remunerations to a Medicare or Medicaid beneficiary that (s)he knows or should know is likely to influence the patient when choosing a health care provider or service that Medicare or Medicaid will pay for in part or full. As such, providers offering telehealth technology to patients must evaluate whether these tools will count as remunerations in violation of the CMP law. Exceptions to the CMP include gifts of nominal value given to patients, promotions to incentivize preventable care activities, and certain co-pay assistance.

OIG Advisory Opinions

The Office of Inspector General (OIG) is principally charged with enforcing the Federal fraud and abuse laws. As such, the OIG publishes opinions to help entities determine whether proposed arrangements would subject them to civil or criminal liability. The OIG has released several advisory opinions expressing its stance on telehealth matters. In 2003, the OIG concluded that providing free medical-alert pagers and an accompanying monitoring system to home health services patients was not an improper inducement under the Civil Monetary Penalties. Instead, the OIG agreed with CMS that these types of telehealth technologies help provide efficient, higher quality care. More recently in 2011, the OIG evaluated arrangements under which a neuro-emergency center at a top-ranked hospital provided telehealth services to community hospitals. The OIG concluded this arrangement would not result in an improper inducement.

State Laws and Telehealth Considerations

In addition to federal Stark, AKS, and CMP laws, telehealth programs are also subject to state fraud and abuse laws. Some states merely integrate the federal laws into their state Medicaid statutes with the same or varying safe harbors and exceptions.

Other states, however, have promulgated rules that expand the scope of the federal laws to apply to private payers. As such, an arrangement that is permissible under federal law may still violate state fraud and abuse laws.

Consistent with the spirit of the federal fraud and abuse laws, many states explicitly prohibit patient brokering. Patient brokering is the illegal practice of a health care entity paying a fee to an individual for bringing them new patients. This practice preys on the vulnerable by inhibiting their freedom to choose a health care provider. Patient brokering has been particularly rampant in the addiction treatment industry. Similarly, some states also have laws prohibiting fee splitting among practitioners who refer patients to each other. As such, telehealth practices should be careful in their efforts to recruit new business not to run afoul of established lines of legal behavior.

Summary for Telehealth Legal and Regulatory Considerations

While there are extensive legal and regulatory considerations that must be considered and addressed during telehealth service development and implementation, these can be readily addressed with appropriate due diligence and input from professionals with requisite expertise. In general, payers—federal, state, and commercial—are coming to recognize the important role telehealth can play with regard to improving overall quality of care. Thus, expending the needed research from a regulatory vantage point is time and effort well spent.

References

1. Ala. Admin. Code 540-X-16.
2. 32 Tex. Admin. Code § 172.12.
3. Virginia Code § 54.1–2901(A)(7).
4. Minn. Stat. §147.032.
5. Conn. Gen. Stat. § 20–9(d).
6. Iowa Admin. Code r. 653–9.1.
7. Mich. Comp. Laws § 333.16171(e).
8. Ala. Code § 34–24–501(a)(3).
9. IMLC.org. [Internet]. [Place unknown]: Interstate Medical Licensure Compact; [cited 2020 June 29]. Available from: https://www.imlcc.org/.
10. Telehealth Services, 42 C.F.R. § 410.78(a)(3) (2001).
11. 10–144 CMR, Chapter 101, MaineCare Benefits Manual, Chapter I, Section 4.06–2(B) (June 15, 2020).
12. Board Opinion Regarding the Use of Telemedicine Technologies in the Practice of Medicine: Ky. Bd. of Md. Licensure. June 19, 2014. Available from: https://kbml.ky.gov/board/Documents/Board%20Opinion%20regarding%20The%20Use%20of%20Telemedicine%20Technologies%20in%20the%20Practice%20of%20Medicine.pdf.
13. Practicing Medicine Through Telehealth Technology: Ca. Bd. of Med. [cited 2020 June 29]. Available from: http://www.mbc.ca.gov/Licensees/Telehealth.aspx.

14. Ca. Bus. & Prof. Code § 2290.5.
15. 1 Tex. Admin. Code § 354.1432(3)(B).
16. 1 Tex. Admin. Code § 279.16(g)(3).
17. Iowa Admin. Code r. 653–13.11(14).
18. Iowa Admin. Code r. 653–13.11(7)(b)(3).
19. Iowa Admin. Code r. 653–13.11(8).
20. COVID-19 Information Page. United States Department of Justice, Drug Enforcement Administration. 2020. https://www.deadiversion.usdoj.gov/coronavirus.html. Accessed 29 June 2020.
21. Ind. Code, § 25–1-9.5–8.
22. Implementation of the Ryan Haight Online Pharmacy Consumer Protection Act of 2008. Fed Regist [regulation on the Internet]. 2009 April 6 [cited June 28 2020]; 74:15596. Available from: https://www.federalregister.gov/documents/2013/07/01/2013-15596/privacy-act-implementation.
23. Improving Access to Remote Behavioral Health Treatment Act, S. 2, 115th Cong. (2018).
24. Code of Medical Ethics, Opinion 1.1.1. Patient-Physician Relationship. American Medical Association. https://www.ama-assn.org/delivering-care/patient-physician-relationships. Accessed 28 June 2020.
25. Ala. Code, § 34–22–83(c).
26. Cal. Bus. & Prof. Code, § 2290.5.
27. Fla. Admin. Code, r. 64B8–9.0141.
28. Board Opinion Regarding the Use of Telemedicine Technologies in the Practice of Medicine. Ky. Bd. of Md. Licensure. 2014.
29. Position Statement: Contact with Patients Before Prescribing. N.C. Med. Bd. 2015.
30. Position Statement: Telemedicine. N.C. Med. Bd. 2014.
31. Id. Code, § 54–5705.
32. Medicare and Medicaid Programs: Changes Affecting Hospital and Critical Access Hospital Conditions of Participation: Telemedicine Credentialing and Privileging. Fed Regist [regulation on the Internet]. 2011 May 5 [cited June 28 2020]; 76:25550. Available from: https://www.federalregister.gov/documents/2011/05/05/2011-10875/medicare-and-medicaid-programs-changes-affecting-hospital-and-critical-access-hospital-conditions-of-.
33. Medicare and Medicaid Programs: Proposed Changes Affecting Hospital and Critical Access Hospital (CAH) Conditions of Participation (CoPs): Credentialing and Privileging of Telemedicine Physicians and Practitioners. Fed Regist [regulation on the Internet]. 2010 May 26 [cited June 28 2020]; 75 FR 29479. Available from: https://www.federalregister.gov/documents/2010/05/26/2010-12647/medicare-and-medicaid-programs-proposed-changes-affecting-hospital-and-critical-access-hospital-cah.
34. Condition of Participation: Medical Staff, 42 C.F.R. § 482.22 (1986).
35. Limitation on Certain Physician Referrals 42 U.S.C. § 1395nn (1935).
36. Criminal Penalties for Acts Involving Federal Health Care Programs 42 U.S.C. § 1320a-7b (1935).
37. Exceptions, 42 C.F.R. § 1001.952(x), (y) (1992).
38. Civil Monetary Penalties 42 U.S.C. § 1320a-7a(a) (1935).

Chapter 3
Telehealth Finance Variables and Successful Business Models

Bryan T. Arkwright, Monica L. Nash, and Morgan E. Light

Introduction

Successful telehealth business models are a topic of regular discussion in the healthcare industry, and the financial details of telehealth programs, initiatives, and companies are at the center of the debate [1]. The goal for this chapter is to define and articulate the financial variables and business models that are the lifeblood of today's successful telehealth programs. The financial and business models surrounding telehealth are unique for a number of reasons [1], principally because the calculations and architecture of such models often contain many continuous variables [2].

The continuous variables of telehealth finance and business models include the following: people (clinical providers and patients), geography (rural or a metropolitan areas), telehealth governance structure, the service provided, the reimbursement or coverage eligibility, the technology used, the quality of care rendered, and the outcome of the care rendered. These continuous variables can make it challenging to actuate financial sustainability and determine if or when a telehealth program, initiative, or company has a successful business model. "In any case, health care

B. T. Arkwright (✉)
School of Law, Wake Forest University, Winston-Salem, NC, USA

Cromford Health, Charlotte, NC, USA

Partners in Digital Health/Telehealth and Medicine Today Journal, New York, NY, USA
e-mail: arkwribt@wfu.edu; bryan@cromfordhealth.com

M. L. Nash
Department of eHealth, SCP Health, Mobile, AL, USA

M. E. Light
Department of Surgical Intensive Care, Wake Forest Baptist Medical Center, Winston-Salem, NC, USA

© Springer Nature Switzerland AG 2021
D. W. Ford, S. R. Valenta (eds.), *Telemedicine*, Respiratory Medicine,
https://doi.org/10.1007/978-3-030-64050-7_3

managers facing a decision must deal with the phenomenon known as bounded rationality, or the limits imposed on decision making by costs, human abilities and errors, time, technology, and the tractability of data," asserts Yasar Ozcan [3]. Telehealth adds another layer of complexity on top of an industry that already has data tractability challenges due to the nature of data being generated and collected at two distinct locations – patient side and clinical provider side. Traditional business models in industries outside of healthcare have more defined, stable, and tractable data inputs and outputs.

Telehealth Governance and Investment

Telehealth governance is defined as the management structure for advancing a telehealth strategy by ensuring that the telehealth program has the intentional leadership and investment to achieve an expected performance level or business model expectation.

Establishing governance is an essential first step toward reaching a consensus on how best to define, track, and organize the telehealth financial variables for a successful business model. Inherent to a successful telehealth business model is strong governance with a responsibility and accountability of intentional leadership focused on three key functions: management, prioritization of services, and achieving return on investment or value on investment [4].

Focusing first on management, it is integral to demonstrate telehealth leadership capability in the following ways:

- Telehealth leadership provides the telehealth stakeholders timely, thorough, relevant, and accurate information about the telehealth industry.
- Telehealth leadership provides telehealth stakeholders information regarding the market in which it operates and how its strategies and operations support and strengthen the overall strategic and financial plans.

Telehealth leadership is most recognizable industry wide in the form of a Telehealth Executive Champion and a Primary Telehealth Leader. Telehealth Executive Champions are identified by individuals serving in existing senior leadership roles including but not limited to:

- Chief Information Officer
- Chief Technology Officer
- Chief Executive Officer
- Chief Operating Officer
- Chief Medical Officer
- Chief Medical Information Officer
- Chief Human Resources Officer

Primary Telehealth Leaders are identified by individuals serving in leadership roles including but not limited to:

- Senior Vice President
- Chief Telehealth Officer
- Vice President
- Executive Director
- Director of Telehealth
- Medical Director
- Administrator, Manager
- Coordinator

Telehealth organizational structures are necessary to support the Primary Telehealth Leader and Executive Champions to achieve a successful telehealth business model. A top priority of the Telehealth Executive Champion and the Telehealth Leader is formation of a multidisciplinary team of clinical and administrative leaders to serve on an executive and/or steering committee for telehealth. An example of the departments represented on a telehealth executive and/or steering committee includes the following [4]:

- Business Development
- Clinical Engineering/Biomedical
- Clinical Operations
- Compliance/Risk Management
- Finance
- Innovation
- IT/IS (information technology/information systems)
- Legal
- Marketing
- Medical Staff/Medical Affairs
- Nursing
- Philanthropy
- Population Health
- Quality
- Revenue Cycle

A multidisciplinary telehealth executive and/or steering committee should execute the following core responsibilities:

- Establish policies and procedures for developing, operating, recruiting, and compensating all key telehealth stakeholders involved. This includes, but is not limited to:

  - Clinical providers
  - Full and part-time support staff
  - Medical director leadership dedicated to telehealth

- Evaluate key performance indicator dashboards of actual results against plans according to operations, clinical, technical, and financial goals

Telehealth governance effectiveness can be evaluated by assessing seven key needs of the multidisciplinary telehealth executive and/or steering committee (as directed by the telehealth leader and executive champion) [4] (derived from White and Griffith's *Well Managed Healthcare Organization*):

1. Meet legal requirements; licensing across state and international lines, credentialing at facilities and payers, coding, billing, reimbursement, hardware and software, security, CMS (Centers for Medicare & Medicaid Services), JCAHO (Joint Commission on Accreditation of Healthcare Organizations), and state, country-specific departments of health and human services
2. Compliance, policies, and procedures that back-up and align with legal requirements
3. Continuing education
4. Use of dashboards and automated data tracking
5. Culture
6. Conflicts of interest
7. Telehealth ROI performance (i.e., clinical, operational, financial, technical)

Telehealth investment is a direct by-product of intentional leadership and telehealth governance. The investment is in the leadership and organizational structure to fund and finance programs, strategies, and operating budgets. Several illustrative organizational structures are shown in Figs. 3.1 and 3.2.

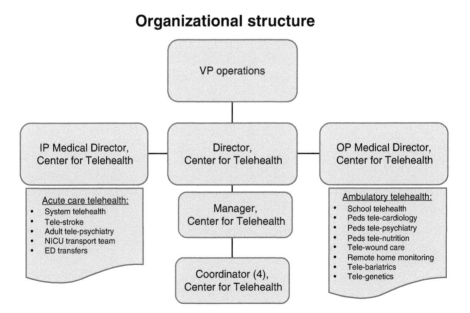

Fig. 3.1 Organizational structure in which all department telehealth programs report to the Center for Telehealth Director and the VP of Operations. (Medium-sized eight (8) hospital health system in the Southeast) [4]

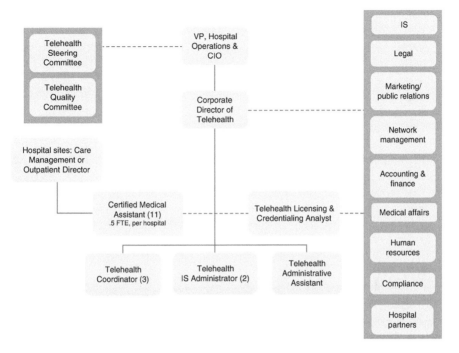

Fig. 3.2 Organizational structure with shared reporting to either the VP, Hospital Operations, and CIO or the Corporate Director of Telehealth. Ultimately, all departments are under control of the VP, Hospital Operations, and CIO. (Large-sized twenty plus (20+) hospital international health system) [4]

Using Governance to Prioritize Telehealth Investment

Ongoing review and prioritization of telehealth services complements telemedicine governance and the appropriate and aligned investment to operating and capital budgets. This includes starting new programs, as well as prioritizing or vetoing recommendations to optimize and expand services. A proven approach is assessment, with consideration of a defined organizational telehealth methodology.

Methodology used by telehealth programs to prioritize investment includes but is not limited to the following:

- *Clinical value*: Implementing the telehealth program significantly improves patient experience and access, while reducing cost and improving quality.
- *Physician/provider engagement*: A physician or provider champion candidate is present with significant buy-in from colleagues in the clinical discipline. A strong team and team lead are present with a lead backup.
- *Administrative support*: Senior leadership supports and validates the physician or provider champion and the clinical discipline's strength for successful implementation. Appropriate legal and risk counsel has been contacted.

- *Strategic plan congruence*: The clinical discipline and the telehealth program align with the organization's strategic plan.
- *Access to funding and technology*: The clinical discipline, or if present, tele-health office/department, has access to funding (organizational funding/capital, federal grant, industry grant, foundation/association grant, or other). Technology may exist or new technology investment may be required. The initiative's reim-bursement, ROI, and VOI are understood.
- *Clinical capacity*: The clinical discipline has the capacity (i.e., time and man-power) for successful implementation short term and long term (1, 3, and 5 years). Implementing impacts capacity for the clinical discipline in a positive and manageable way.
- *Operational and logistical complexity*: Ease of implementation does not pose major operational barriers. Pre-work may or may not be accomplished to date.

Telehealth Finance Variables

As telehealth programs establish their leadership structures and governance for tele-health, they can mature to a higher level of operational excellence through aware-ness of the available telehealth finance variables. A total of 16 telehealth financial variables are defined in Table 3.1 [4–7]. All or a portion of the listed telehealth finance variables can be identified and tracked for telehealth purposes.

Awareness of the breadth of telehealth finance variables is essential to the opera-tions of successful telehealth programs, initiatives, and companies. Furthermore, the laws and regulations of US states, US federal initiatives, and additional coun-tries and states outside the United States create major confusion across stakeholders in the industry. A lack of defined standards and varied definitions of industry terms, business models, and financing mechanisms is a significant impediment. Confusion is often a by-product of an industry experiencing rapid growth or major innovation, and telehealth continues to see movement in both each year. A review of state and federal laws and regulations can be found in Chap. 2.

Compound the lack of industry standards with the number of active players in the industry, and one can quickly feel overwhelmed by the logistics of developing suc-cessful telehealth programs [8]. One substantial barrier is a general lack of knowl-edge needed to appropriately utilize telehealth codes and comply with payer requirements for billing and reimbursement. Navigating the payer landscape has several notable compliance and financial sustainability challenges:

- Improper documentation for telehealth services
- Improper payments for telehealth services
- Missed opportunities to collect revenue
- Missed opportunities for cost savings

In calendar year 2016, Medicare paid a total of $28,748,210 for telehealth ser-vices, spread across a total of 496,396 claims. This includes payments to distant site

Table 3.1 Telehealth finance variables and definitions

Telehealth finance variables	Definition
Fee-for-service (FFS) payments	Defined as reimbursement (payment) for a telehealth service based on a determined or negotiated fee schedule that is not tied to quality of the patient care delivered or a desired patient outcome. The fee is paid if and how often the service is delivered and is centered around the volume of the service delivered. Growing the service increases revenue with no correlated connection to patient and provider satisfaction or quality and outcomes. The healthcare industry is moving away from fee-for service reimbursement models. Numerous payers in the healthcare industry and varying state-specific telehealth laws and regulations create a widely varied range of fees and services covered, creating inconsistency for tracking and reporting by telehealth programs. Common fee-for-service payers include Medicare, State Medicaid, Private Payers, and Self Pay.
Value-based payments	Defined as reimbursement (payment) for a telehealth service dependent on the cost, efficiency, quality, and outcome. The fee is paid if and how the service is deemed to be of value to the patient, and is centered around the quadruple AIM of cost, quality, clinician experience, and access or population health [5]. Telehealth can be a cornerstone of value-based payments, as it can maximize access to care in an efficient manner. However, exact financial costs associated with value-based payments are not standardized in the industry, so assigning a financial value to telehealth as part of a value-based payment is varied or continuously measured until defined by the telehealth program.
Per member per month	Defined as reimbursement (payment) for a telehealth service that is associated with the ongoing availability of a service to a patient or group of patients or as part of an extended care plan where care is delivered on a regular basis at least once a month or more. Per member per month reimbursement is common among telehealth programs who utilize the Center for Medicare and Medicaid Services (CMS)/Medicare Chronic Condition Management (CCM), Transitional Care Management (TCM), and Remote Patient Monitoring (RPM) codes and reimbursement. One example is using a RPM initiative that reimburses the hospital per patient per month in an effort to reduce 30-day hospital readmissions. The revenue and savings in this example is both direct and indirect in how it presents to the hospital or health system. Per member per month reimbursement is also common among telehealth companies who offer large and small employer groups access to a telehealth consult service.
Coinsurance	Defined as reimbursement (payment) for a portion (percentage) of the cost of a telehealth service or a determined or negotiated fee schedule based on a service category.
Shared savings	Defined as reimbursement (payment) as part of a determined or negotiated outcome or quality benchmark being achieved for a defined population through a telehealth service, can be reimbursed on a rolling or set schedule (often quarterly or annually). One party agrees to pay a telehealth program, initiative, or company an agreed-upon payment at a particular quality benchmark or expected outcome. Achieving the quality benchmark or expected outcome saves a party an expected cost and they in turn pay the telehealth program a portion of that cost savings.

(continued)

Table 3.1 (continued)

Telehealth finance variables	Definition
Reduced readmissions	Defined as the avoidance of readmitting patients to a hospital in less than 30 days utilizing telehealth. Hospitals and health systems are subjected to losing their collected revenue for an inpatient CMS (Medicare) stay if that patient returns to any hospital and is readmitted for any reason in 30 days or less. The loss of revenue associated with these patients on an annual cycle can be significant and jeopardize the entire health system or hospital's financial viability. Utilization of telehealth to work with at-risk patients and populations is intended to reduce this annual cost and be a measurable savings for the hospital or health system.
Patient satisfaction	Defined as the satisfaction a patient has with telehealth. Telehealth services are convenient, centered around the patient, and improve the access to a range of specialists. Measuring the satisfaction of a telehealth patient and the correlated financial benefit to both the patient and the health system is a continuous variable to note, albeit complex to define a standard.
Avoidable patient days	Defined as the difference in the count of days a patient has in an inpatient setting if they have access to a qualified specialist provided via a telehealth compared to not having that access. Having timely and efficient access to services such as neurology and psychiatry consults as an example can result in the reduction of avoidable patient days, creating a cost savings for the hospital [4, 6].
Avoidable visits to emergency department	Defined as the count of visits an emergency department has for patients who did not have emergent needs for care. Telehealth can reduce avoidable visits to the emergency department by giving patients a convenient and accessible option to receive care by a qualified medical professional.
Provider time (efficiency)	Defined as the time a provider spends with a patient via telehealth. Depending on a hospital or health system's regional facilities, providers who use telehealth may experience an increase in time spent with patients due to a decrease in need to drive to multiple sites to see patients. Maximizing provider time with clinical care can make providers more efficient if part of a well-designed and managed business model.
Capacity & resource utilization	Defined as the capacity and utilization of resources or assets associated with telehealth. The hardware, software, and technical personnel associated with telehealth have a cost. Tracking that cost with the utilization ensures this continuous variable can be optimized and allocated accurately against monthly, quarterly, and annual budgets.
Total cost of care and quality of care	Defined as a patient's total or episodic cost of care associated with telehealth when compared to the total cost of care associated with comparative in-person care. Evaluating the quality of care and patient outcomes associated with telehealth compared to in-person care is important to determine ongoing value and sustainability of telehealth.
Downstream referral revenue	Defined as the referrals and associated revenue that can accompany a telehealth program. A telehealth service is often establishing a market presence (either online or through a remote or affiliate clinic or hospital site) in an area or region where there is not a physical presence. In addition to the patients served directly through telehealth, those patients may continue to seek additional in-person services or additional online services. Without the presence and initial access promulgated by telehealth, the downstream referrals and increase in services from patients in that region would not have been realized.

Table 3.1 (continued)

Telehealth finance variables	Definition
Downstream ancillary revenue	Defined as the ancillary revenue (imaging, drugs, hospital admissions revenue, reduced transfers revenue) that can accompany telehealth. The new presence of a previously unavailable specialist type due to telehealth can increase the ancillary revenue of an inpatient unit, emergency department, or clinic through increased testing, treatments, hospitalization, and emergency department visits.
Facility fees	Defined as the reimbursement (payment) when a telehealth patient presents to a qualifying healthcare site; there is a code (Q3014) that can be utilized by the qualifying sites and it is recognized by public and private payers. Successful telehealth business models leverage this reimbursement within their network despite the low amount of associated reimbursement per encounter.
Extramural funding	Defined as the extramural or outside funding to a telehealth program. Extramural funding is common in telehealth and is derived from various sources and motives. Extramural funding includes federal grants, federal pilot and demonstration programs (Centers for Medicare and Medicaid Services, Agency for Healthcare Research and Quality, Health Resources and Services Administration, United States Department of Agriculture, National Institutes of Health); state-sponsored legislative initiatives (South Carolina, Mississippi, Florida, North Carolina); private or endowment grant programs; and venture capital or private equity investment. Federal, state, and private or endowment-centered grant programs are designed to assist with the startup and launch cost of a telehealth program, often targeting regional areas with identified healthcare provider and access needs [7]. Since its inception, the USDA Distance Learning and Telehealth Grant has funded numerous programs across the United States and Territories since it started in 1995. Venture capital and private equity investment into telehealth has increased year over year since the late 1990s, often targeting high growth potential companies with a vision to improve healthcare on a regional and global scale. A key similarity of the types of extramural funding is that in every situation, predetermined or negotiated plans and expectations are set with clear accountabilities and responsibilities to achieve by the involved stakeholders. A key difference of the types of extramural funding is the element of generating sales or value on the side of venture capital and private equity investment, whereas grant and federal funding often require reporting on the achieved healthcare access and clinical results or outcomes. Successful telehealth business models will seek and compete for extramural funding as appropriate and when it aligns with the mission, vision, and values of the telehealth program.

providers and originating site payments. Compare this amount to the previous year (2015), in which Medicare paid a total of $22,449,968 for telehealth services, spread across a total of 372,518 claims [7]. Note that the figures are slightly different than reported in prior years, as CMS changed its data collection and calculation methodology in this time window.

The change from 2015 to 2016 realized a 33% increase in the number of Medicare telehealth claims submitted and a 28% increase in total payments. This uptick in total payments is not attributable to fee schedule rate increases, but rather to more providers using telehealth services with their traditional Medicare fee-for-service beneficiaries [9].

The major increases in utilization and submission of telehealth claims during the last few years are as follows [9]. Notable increase from 2015 to 2016 shows a trend expected to continue. The Office of Inspector General (OIG) and the Center for Medicare and Medicaid Services announced in the Fall of 2016 that due to the significant increase in claims and payments in 2016, they would be actively auditing programs for compliant operations in 2018 and moving forward [10]. Early 2018 brought the first glimpse of activity from the OIG and CMS when they announced they had completed early internal audits on paid claims and found that of 100 audited claims, 31 were identified as non-compliant and against federal and/or state regulations [11]. A breakdown of the audit showed that a majority were related to beneficiaries receiving services at non-rural originating sites. This was followed by claims submitted by ineligible providers and an assortment of other violations in single-digit numbers.

Many important changes to federal regulations were implemented with regard to telehealth billing as part of the government's response to the COVID-19 pandemic. Some of the more significant changes included removing the restrictions on the patient location and allowing telehealth to be provided in the home, expanding the list of covered services and eligible providers, and establishing a waiver to allow physicians to practice across state lines. Whether these policy changes will be sustained remains to be seen. Additional interim rules such as the HIPAA flexibility on the use of telehealth platforms are expected to return to the traditional policy post-pandemic [12].

The key factors that can impact telehealth billing and reimbursement requirements include but are not limited to:

- Eligible providers
- Eligible services
- Eligible locations, sites of service (geography)
- Covered codes, CMS
- Place of Service (POS) Code 02 (to indicate telehealth requirements were met)
- Federal and state legislation
- Commercial payer contracting and negotiating (state or nationally applicable)

Successful Telehealth Business Models

A successful telehealth business model begins with the knowledge of financial variables and ends with organized and efficient operations. A successful telehealth business model will demonstrate the following attributes:

- Safe – The care is equal to or better than traditional in person care for the use case/clinical service.
- Appropriate – The care provided is appropriate for the patient's needs [4].
- Patient Centered – The care and services provided are focused on the patient's needs during and after the visit concludes.

- User Friendly – Patients, providers, and caregivers can easily navigate the hardware, software, and interfaces involved before, during, and after the visit concludes.
- Compliant – The telehealth program's care and providers are meeting all federal and state laws and regulations.
- Mission Driven/Strategically Aligned – Key safety, clinical, economic/financial, sociocultural, and other goals are defined, tracked, and align within the telehealth program's ownership and operations [4].
- Value – The "Value Proposition" measures the total benefit attained from using telehealth. In healthcare, the IHI (Institute for Healthcare Improvement) advocated a "triple aim" of value: the patient experience, improving the health of populations, and cost of care. Telehealth can contribute to each of these key dimensions.

Telehealth business models are closely tied to telehealth mode/type of delivery and both are an ongoing evolution in the healthcare industry. The most prevalent and successful business models will identify with one of the eight telehealth delivery modes shown in Table 3.2 [11, 13–19].

Table 3.2 Telehealth business models

Telehealth mode	Definition	Patient interaction
Direct-to-consumer (patient): urgent care access, primary care oriented	A patient driven, on-demand telehealth service. Access to the service will be focused on clinical services that can be completed without an additional clinical staff member or provider being with the patient, thus the service is direct to the patient or consumer [11, 13].	The patient may become aware of the service on their own and request a telehealth visit or the patient may become aware of the service as being part of their employer's health plan, and access may be fully covered or partially covered by their health insurance.
Organization to organization	A telehealth program, initiative, or company contracts with a healthcare provider to provide a specific clinical service. The service may be a contracted fee per consult or subscription based service based on a defined or estimated utilization.	The patient will become aware of the service while they are being cared for by the healthcare provider in an emergent setting, inpatient setting, or outpatient setting. (Stroke, neurology, and mental health are most prevalent)
Clinician to clinician	A telehealth program, initiative, or company contracts with a healthcare provider to provide a peer-to-peer specialty consulting service for difficult and/or specialty cases.	The patient may or may not be aware of the service while they are being cared for by the healthcare provider who utilizes a clinician-to-clinician video model, as some utilize with patient present and others do not.

(continued)

Table 3.2 (continued)

Telehealth mode	Definition	Patient interaction
Continuous remote monitoring for intensive care unit (ICU) patients or tele-ICU	Tele-ICU programs provide continuous remote oversight for patients in monitored ICUs from a central operations center staffed by a multidisciplinary ICU team [14, 15].	Patients and families are aware of the tele-ICU as each room is outfitted with emergency buttons and two-way communications. These programs typically include robust data tracking and reporting for quality measures and ROI.
Online patient access/portals/technology: second opinions and HIT portals	A telehealth program contracts with a healthcare provider to provide a second opinion service through online/web-based asynchronous access to a clinical provider [14, 16–19].	The patient may become aware of the service through their primary care provider or the healthcare provider they utilize for the majority of their care, by provider referral, or by individual searching.
mHealth/medical apps: self-tracking apps, diagnostics, care support	A telehealth program contracts with a healthcare provider or patient to provide a mobile-oriented application for healthcare or care support; may be in the form of remote patient monitoring for chronic disease management.	The patient will be aware of the service through individual searching or may have mHealth (mobile health) software, and/or an application prescribed to them by their healthcare provider.
Hardware/software: telehealth equipment, software, robots, carts, tablets	A telehealth program contracts with a telehealth company for equipment, hardware (robots, carts, tablets) or software.	The patient will be aware of the equipment, hardware, or software when the patient is having the telehealth encounter in a home, healthcare clinic, or hospital location.
International: US to another country telehealth	A US telehealth program contracts with an international entity to provide care from one country to another.	The patient will become aware of the service while they are being cared for by the healthcare provider in an emergent setting, inpatient setting, or outpatient setting.

Additional telehealth business and care delivery models will continue to emerge as the industry evolves. Every telehealth business and care delivery model involves patient care, and it is important to keep the seven attributes of successful telehealth business models in mind when interacting with telehealth. Each telehealth business model can benefit from having a clear and defined contract of all terms and responsibilities of each party involved. The negotiation, drafting, and execution process of clear and defined telehealth contracts are important cornerstones of success when designing and operating a successful telehealth business model.

Return on Investment (ROI) and Value on Investment (VOI)

Universal adoption of telehealth continues to lag despite improved technology and increasing amounts of evidence demonstrating effectiveness. Two key reasons for lagging adoption include the following [20]:

- Complexity of policy at both a federal and state level related to reimbursement for telehealth services.
- The fragmented approach that organizations are using to forecast return on investment (ROI), creating a bleak picture of financial returns and thus program feasibility.

Traditional business models within healthcare focus on direct revenue gained primarily through fee-for-service reimbursement. Approaching telehealth through a fee-for-service lens as the dominant input to return on investment (ROI) is flawed in that it excludes some of the key benefits and underlying value of telehealth program such as cost, quality, efficiency and access, which will be referred to in this chapter as value on investment (VOI). Unlike traditional return on investment models, financial benefits in healthcare also come in the form of cost avoidance and downstream revenue opportunities. Telehealth evaluations will need to deploy varied methods and approaches to estimate telehealth ROI, thinking more broadly in terms of how telehealth functions as an asset by generating value in the form of cost savings, increased efficiency, and downstream revenue opportunity.

Deploying varied methods and approaches to analyzing telehealth ROI and VOI will require creating business models within frameworks that include a variety of financial inputs. The use of a variety of financial inputs will generate a more complete picture of all financial gains and cost savings associated with telehealth efforts. The nuances and challenges of measuring ROI and VOI and the evolving field of health economics is such an important topic that it prompted the organization of the 2016 Global Health Economics Consortium Colloquium co-sponsored by leading researchers and faculty at Stanford Health Policy, UCSF Global Health Sciences, and the UC Berkeley School of Public Health [21].

A Departure from Volume to Value

Traditionally, the business case for telehealth is based on fee-for-service revenue collected from insurers or patients and viewed as the key input to project ROI. As the landscape of healthcare transitions from volume and direct revenue to a system focused on quality, access and cost, the need to adapt financial practices estimating return and value associated must evolve. New structures and programs including Accountable Care Organizations and CMS codes that recognize virtual check-ins are sparking development and advancement to understanding and articulating the telehealth return and value on investment [22].

Traditional return on investment can be thought of as the gain from the investment, or revenue, minus the cost of the investment, which yields net profit, divided by the cost of the investment:

$$\text{Traditional ROI} = (\text{total revenue} - \text{total cost}) \text{ OR net profit} / \text{total cost}$$

The problem with this calculation in today's evolving healthcare environment is that the "Total Revenue" input is driven by fee-for-service, or volume-based, payments. Telehealth value on investment must be thought of more broadly from a financial perspective to include all contributions translating to benefit for the organization. Currently, most of the technology costs and the consultations carried out through telemedicine are not reimbursed and motivation is typically either through improving system efficiency and/or external funding [1]. Return on investment is flexible and can be modified to support the industry or situation. In the case of healthcare, benefit (direct and indirect) is a key element of the return on investment expression. What is included in the telehealth VOI will vary organization to organization and program to program and may include avoidable cost, shared savings, and referrals to the sponsoring institution. Value on investment can be thought of as the gain from the investment, in terms of revenue (direct), cost savings (indirect), downstream revenue (indirect) and increased efficiencies (indirect), minus the cost of the investment, which yields net value, divided by the cost of the investment:

$$\text{VOI} = (\text{total direct revenue} + \text{total indirect revenue OR cost savings}) - \text{total cost}$$

Key Concepts of Telehealth ROI and VOI

Defining a financial ROI for a telehealth service or program may require considering new inputs that translate to returns in the form of value, or VOI, yielding benefit and goodwill that can be translated to financial realization, in addition to profits. Some of the core intangible benefits that may translate to returns in the form of VOI include the following:

- Eliminates geographical boundaries to leverage distributed clinical expertise and capacity
- Improves quality of life for the patient and family
- Enables opportunities to further extend care to new market areas and international locations
- Provides new collaboration methods to enable new partnerships
- Improves the ability to collaborate among physicians, departments, locations, and services to make more informed patient care decisions and coordinated care delivery
- Provides opportunity to deliver care more efficient and better manage care transitions

One metaphorical approach to the process is to brainstorm financial inputs as one would view an iceberg. There will be inputs that are on or above the surface that translate directly to profits and can be quantified rather precisely, such as fee-for-service revenue and copays. There will also be inputs that are below the surface that translate more indirectly and may be more difficult or less precisely quantified numerically, such as reduced readmissions, increased provider efficiency, and increased referrals to the system. It is common to define a mix of variables that can be broken apart, evaluated, and fit into a mix of complimentary financial levers that create a compelling business case. Figure 3.3 is one example of the iceberg analogy used to project returns and value for a telehealth program, initiative, or company [23].

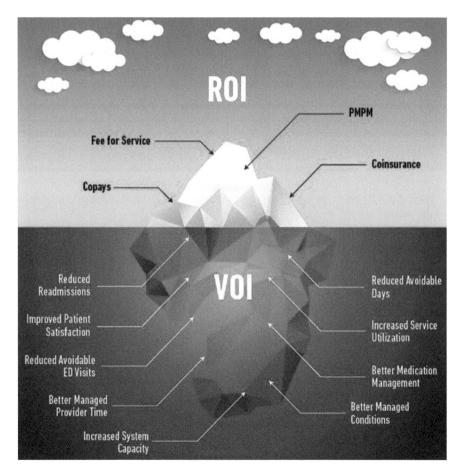

Fig. 3.3 Iceberg analogy depicting the value of telehealth, specifically remote patient monitoring, is both clear and direct or above the service, but also includes below the surface value that is still important in the design and calculation of impact, quality, ROI, VOI, and overall program or project sustainability

Exploring "Above the Surface" Inputs

The practice of building an ROI for telehealth is fluid and continuous, and associated inputs will likely evolve as the industry releases innovative programs, technologies, and ways of doing business. Direct revenue streams, referred to on the iceberg as "above the surface," may be revenue in the form of fee-for-service, site-of-service facility fees or hospital billing, and direct to patient payments. If requirements are appropriately planned for and met, fee-for-service revenue can be the least complex ROI input to forecast. Below is an exploration of "Above the Surface" inputs that may be a part of a telehealth program:

- *Fee-for-Service (Professional Billing)* is reimbursement from eligible telehealth codes with affixed modifiers, such as GT, GQ, or 95, for telehealth services. Professional, or fee-for-service, payments within telehealth must meet rules and requirements of payers.

  As of the 2018, Medicare reimburses for 97 different CPT and HCPCS codes at an average rate of $115–125 per code, with Medicaid and private payers in many states matching or exceeding that number of covered codes. To be eligible for payment and in compliance with payer requirements, telehealth programs should consult insurer policies for telehealth and telehealth reimbursement. The landscape continues to evolve and become more favorable to payment; however, many payers still have conditions for payment related to rurality, providers, documentation, and services. In 2019, Medicare, which is one of the more restrictive payers for telehealth services, lifted the geography restriction for payment for telehealth services for telestroke, which is a strong favorable signal to the industry [22].
- *Site-of-Service Facility Fee (Hospital Billing)* is reimbursement paid to the site where the patient is located during the time of telehealth service. It is known within Medicare as the Originating Site Facility Fee and identified by eligible code Q3014 by many payers. Facility Fee payments range from $15 to $40 per encounter. If the site of service is part of a larger system or organization, this payment should be considered as part of the direct revenue stream of a telehealth program, initiative, or company [22]. To obtain specific information on the eligible code and rate reimbursed, consult individual payer policies on a per-state basis.
- *Direct to Patient*, also known as out of pocket or self-pay, is defined as point-of-service payments from direct to consumer programs. It could also be in the form of copayments and/or coinsurance. This form of payment is common in direct to consumer telehealth programs caring for primary and minor acute patient needs. On average, a virtual primary care visit with a direct to patient fee will run between 25 and 75 per visit, for a secure, face-to-face video encounter.
- *Direct Contracting* is a growing trend and occurs when groups such as employers and insurers partner with a provider of telehealth services to receive payment according to a predefined contract. Direct contracting has been referenced by Snap MD CEO, Dave Skibinski, as a telehealth "Trojan Horse" due to the disrup-

tion of the natural flow of referrals that would typically occur within health systems now being directly contracted to vendors [24]. Although the trend has been for telehealth service providers to adopt this business model, hospitals and health systems are many times in a position to also use this financial model. The contracted rate for services is largely dependent on the market and service being offered and may vary greatly from contract to contract.

Exploring "Below the Surface" Inputs

The practice of building a VOI for telehealth goes beyond "above the surface" inputs to draw synergies and net positive impact associated with cost savings and downstream revenue into the overall business case for telehealth programs. Indirect revenue streams, referred to on the iceberg as "below the surface," are more difficult to measure and predict when projecting financial returns for telehealth programs and services, however, are still a vital component of the total telehealth picture. Indirect revenue may come in the form of avoidable cost, economies of scale, quality, and patient satisfaction. Including indirect revenue as part of a telehealth financial model goes beyond return to estimate full value on investment (VOI).

"Organizations across the globe are becoming creative in their approaches to estimating 'below the surface' impact to include as part of a program's VOI. For example, INTEGRIS Health, a self-insured provider, utilizes an advisory committee to evaluate prospective projects and services to work toward establishing metrics to track returns and value. Additionally, new projects require a business plan with a financial ROI and ongoing assessment of clinical and financial performance after launch, according to the eHealth Director, Pam Forducey" [25]. One example is reducing 30-day readmissions using home-based telehealth monitoring equipment. Another is reducing travel expenses for physicians traveling across the state to provide regional outreach. Continued patient engagement is another ROI – particularly for patients who would otherwise not travel long distances for 15–20-minute follow-up visits. For the purposes of this chapter, indirect revenue stream inputs are referred to as the VOI component of a telehealth financial model [25].

Each telehealth program or service will calculate indirect revenue a bit differently. Resources such as case studies and benchmarks are published frequently for a wide range of telehealth specialties and can serve as a starting point for estimating indirect cost savings or revenue generation as part of a telehealth ROI. For example, remote monitoring for chronic care management is an area of telehealth that demonstrates significant indirect revenue opportunity. A study by the Canadian Department of Health and Queens University determined that a remote patient monitoring program yielded a variety of results, which can be translated to data points within a financial model. These included reductions in 911 calls and subsequent paramedic activations, reduced emergency department visits, reduced hospital admissions, and reduced hospital readmissions [26]. Indirect revenue stream inputs

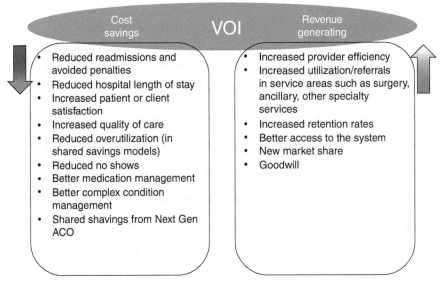

Fig. 3.4 Value on investment visual that lists the cost savings areas of focus and revenue-generating focus areas of telehealth

that should be included to project full VOI within telehealth business cases typically fall into two categories: (1) cost savings and (2) revenue generating. Figure 3.4 highlights possible indirect inputs.

Examples of inputs that could yield cost savings as part of a telehealth program's overall VOI include the following:

- Reduced readmissions and avoided penalties
- Reduced hospital length of stay
- Increased patient or client satisfaction

  - For example, in a recent survey, patients and families who utilized telehealth services felt that it was more convenient than a clinic visit, less disruptive to their life and routine and would choose to use it again [26].

- Increased quality of care
- Reduced overutilization (in shared savings models)

  - For example, a study by Lunney et al. found that in two instances of comparing telehealth to traditional, in-person care a lower rate of hospitalization was reported with telehealth than with traditional, in-person care (2.2 vs. 5.7 days annually per patient). Additionally, another study [27] found that patients utilizing telehealth instead of traditional, in-person care had fewer hospitalizations, shorter length of stay, and fewer visits to the emergency department.

- Reduced no shows

  - For example, a study found that patients who received telehealth were less likely to miss HD treatment sessions compared with patients receiving only standard care [4].

- Better medication management
- Better complex condition management
- Shared shavings from Accountable Care Organization (ACO)
- Avoidable transport costs/miles saved

  - For example, one program found that the average trip travel time from home to clinic was 6.8 hours. Due to the fact that a telehealth visit can avoid unnecessary travel time it saves in transportation costs and time, which can be translated into an average of $486 dollars saved [26].

Examples of inputs that could translate to incremental revenue as part of a telehealth program's overall VOI include the following:

- Increased provider efficiency
- Increased utilization/referrals in service areas such as surgery, ancillary, other specialty services
- Increased retention rates
- Better access to the system
- New market share
- Community goodwill

Challenges to Estimating Telehealth ROI

The promise of strong ROI and VOI for telehealth programs come with unique challenges that should be considered as part of any financial analysis or model. It is also important to consider that since healthcare is so localized, the way in which one program successfully defines and measures telehealth ROI is not necessarily the same as other programs operating in other contexts and environments. Challenges inherent to projecting returns and value on investment in telehealth programs may also widely vary; however, some common issues across the industry include the following:

- Complexities of the healthcare insurance market and payer engagement
- Identifying and quantifying indirect revenue streams
- Measurement and tracking of data in disparate systems

Complexities of the Healthcare Insurance Market and Payer Engagement

The reimbursement environment for telehealth by traditional insurance providers is both varied and complex. Policies and conditions for payment are historically quite restrictive at the federal level. Due to the number of payers and the management of health insurance on a state-by-state basis, the industry is faced with no clear or universal way to determine direct payment for telehealth services. Rather, each individual insurance carrier is left to set policy requirements for themselves, leaving those looking to receive reimbursement to build the appropriate workflows within their programs to satisfy a shifting exponential number of rules.

Despite the complex healthcare insurance market as a significant barrier for telehealth, the future is bright, thanks to new payer engagement strategies and new federal structures and payment demonstration and pilot initiatives available. CMS, DHHS, state DHHS groups, and many other private and federal groups are reimbursing and financing for telehealth services, such as in the Next-Generation ACO [28]. In addition, CMS has removed the originating site restrictions of tele-health services for more ACO members in its Medicare Shared Savings Program [29–31].

Whether or not a telehealth program is participating in an organized new pay-ment model or demonstration project, maintaining detailed documentation and the success or failure of reimbursement is critical. It is invaluable for telehealth pro-grams to proactively focus on having documentable actions of beginning and main-taining relationships with all types of payers. Telehealth programs who have realized success with payers are synonymous with establishing a relationship that is trans-parent and continuous, giving payers an awareness of programs, providers, utiliza-tion, and payment expectations for services rendered via telehealth. A common best practice in telehealth is to track monthly the details of reimbursements collected and denied for telehealth services; these actions will inform ongoing discussions of including new services, determining documentation requirements, and denial reme-diations. These actions alone can yield great clarification and development to rede-fine the delivery of care and payment structures, thus breaking down the complexities [32].

Identifying and Quantifying Indirect Revenue Streams

The difficulty of measuring indirect streams of revenue has been reviewed in this chapter. These difficulties can be due to several factors, including challenges iden-tifying indirect variables that have financial impact, no historical data points to pre-dict the future and defining how to measure and monitor variables in a consistent, reliable way. The variables that create indirect impact may vary by type of telehealth program or service being offered. An article by the Advisory Board explores differ-ent motivations and metrics within telehealth programs that complement direct rev-enue and alternatively measure telehealth's effect on program performance [33].

1. *Real-time virtual visits: Protect and diversify your brand*
     Downstream referrals: Ideally, a real-time virtual visit platform does not just guide new patients into the system; it spurs subsequent use of other in-network services. Downstream referral rate and corresponding revenue can measure plat-form contribution to brand loyalty.

- Existing patient retention rates: Real-time virtual visits meet the consumer desire for accessible, on-demand care and may help retain current patients otherwise drawn by cost or convenience elsewhere. Existing patient retention rates assess whether virtual care prevents patient leakage, promoting long-term consumer engagement with your organization.

2. *Asynchronous store-and-forward: Enhance efficiency*

- Time-to-consult fulfillment: The more quickly providers reply and fulfill requests for care guidance, the greater your time savings. To evaluate operational benefits for your asynchronous store-and-forward solution, benchmark time duration between consult request and provider response against less dynamic platforms, such as telephone and in-person visits.
- Diagnostic accuracy: Don't sacrifice quality for expediency. Measure diagnostic accuracy to ensure that your platform both promotes efficiency and consistently resolves presenting conditions.

3. *Remote patient monitoring: Manage your population health enterprise*

- Readmissions rate: By remotely tracking patient status, providers can use remote patient monitoring to intervene when necessary and avoid care escalation. Measure readmissions rate to evaluate how remote patient monitoring programs prevent penalties and keep patients at home.
- Patient adherence to treatment plan: Among patients with chronic conditions or those recovering from surgery, remote patient monitoring platforms frequently include checklists and reminders to help patients follow care instructions. Tracking treatment adherence demonstrates how a program impacts health behavior and positions an organization for downstream cost savings.

Measurement and Tracking Within Disparate Systems

Inputs to financial models may be housed in different systems that need to be integrated to determine the full picture of "value." This reality creates a challenge in the ongoing measurement and monitoring of variables necessary to develop ROI and VOI. Some of these inputs may be more easily measured and tracked than others; however, they still represent significant opportunity within the financial model of a telehealth program. The telehealth ROI includes indirect and direct variables; and telehealth-specific data can be challenging to collect across different healthcare organization information systems (e.g., EHR (electronic health records), video servers, telehealth vendor platforms, remote home monitoring platforms, HR (human resource) systems, financial systems, and more). It may be prudent to consider using automated software to facilitate rapid and ongoing tracking of telehealth ROI and VOI components.

Achieving Success with Telehealth ROI: Best Practices

Analysis of all telehealth financial variables is an exercise that telehealth programs should complete in partnership with leadership, seeking approval of defined inputs to enable the continuous tracking of their ROI through an established governance structure. Once established, the business case around a telehealth program should be created to determine feasibility. Quarterly reports of the strategic telehealth ROI scorecard across clinical, financial, operational, and technical areas should be reviewed. Telehealth ROIs are unique and complex for every organization according to the maturity of the telehealth program.

To understand how to model the mix of possible telehealth finance variables for the ROI, the telehealth program must understand what the variables are (metrics), define how they are measured (measure), and how they will be tracked on an ongoing basis (monitor). Leading healthcare organizations that regularly track and communicate effectiveness create and ensure a strong telehealth culture that grows across the organization.

Within the reimbursement environment, best practice organizations are navigating these challenges using five key success criteria to ensure compliant and optimized telehealth return on investment processes:

1. *Contracts/Agreements*

   - All entities providing telehealth services have a contract or agreement
   - Agreements for those entities clarify all parties obligations
   - Meets 12 standard contractual provisions for telehealth contracts [34]
   - Providers are appropriately credentialed with payers for billing
   - Arrangements capture the full scope of all parties billing/compensation obligations

2. *Policy/Regulatory*

   - Up-to-date on billing and documentation requirements by payer
   - Monitor changing regulations via frequent reviews
   - Maintain compliance at all times with changing regulations/requirements
   - Ability to quickly communicate
   - Agile response to change
   - Negotiate with payers to drive additional coverage

3. *Standard Operating Procedures*

   - Create a formal telehealth development life cycle
   - Define new program start-up process steps
   - Internal policy requiring new program contract or agreement
   - Standardize approach to provisions
   - Internal policy and/or supporting procedures that promote a centralized Telehealth department

4. *Workflow Design*

- Standardized clinical, technical, operational, and financial workflows
- Automated systems (e.g., build)
- Clear roles and accountability
- Use of smart tools and text to increase documentation efficiency
- Integrate requirements into processes and systems
- Continuous focus on ease of use for end-users

5. *Oversight/Reporting*

- Centralized program oversight
- Establish and communicate program governance
- Real-time, automated data and reporting dashboards to drive utilization, documentation accuracy, quality, ROI
- Automated software to facilitate rapid and ongoing tracking of telehealth ROI/VOI
- Maximization of revenue opportunity
- Denials management process
- Full operational transparency

Other Factors That Impact or Contribute to ROI

Telehealth return on investment can be further strengthened using formal planning that aligns with organizational strategic priorities, well-executed marketing and education efforts, and focus on adoption of the model.

Strategic planning of telehealth programs to align project return on investment to market drivers or reasons for starting the program is a key element to successful launch and operations, which will translate to the bottom line. Organizations that take the time to understand the unique needs of their customers and market are at an advantage over those that do not, which can greatly contribute to a program's financial health. Market drivers for telehealth may include the following:

- Shortage of providers and specialty care, particularly in rural or underserved areas
- Rising number of people needing care due to aging populations
- Changing reimbursement landscape focused on management across the continuum of health, rather than single episodes of care
- Shift in the way customers and patients are seeking care, where convenience is expected
- Smart-phone use and the way technology applications support our lifestyles

Along with intentional planning and strategic alignment, telehealth programs will need to consider how they outreach and educate about program offerings to internal and external audiences. Marketing and outreach efforts should go hand in hand with the implementation and ongoing operations of a new program or service. Formal orientation sessions are one way that organizations are reaching out to populations they serve to increase program utilization.

The University of Mississippi Medical Center (UMMC) conducted a pilot study, which identified commonalities of employees who took advantage of UMMC's corporate telehealth services. The study gleaned several key characteristics related to utilization of the corporate telehealth program by their employees. Interestingly, the study determined highest utilization of the program by employees ages of 30–49 years who also attended a formal orientation session. The orientation session was conducted by both the employer's human resources leadership and a UMMC corporate telehealth representative. A key takeaway from this study is that corporations seeking to adopt corporate telehealth services as an effective method to reduce overall healthcare costs and employee absenteeism may further benefit from including a required orientation to the program, while also developing additional methods for outreach and education to employees who would not otherwise seek out medical treatment [11]. Edgerton et al. reviewed the number of e-visits by type of program orientation, type of corporation, and the number of e-visits per 100 enrollees per year [13]. In general, across a wide spectrum of employer types (e.g., banking, manufacturing, education, development), formal orientation was associated with significantly higher rates of employee utilization of the e-visit options. Beyond formal education about program offerings, acceptance of technology is a key concern across the industry. Society continues to increase use of and reliance on video and mobile technologies. The acceptance and growth of telehealth follows that same trajectory; however, it is important to anticipate and understand how to overcome existing barriers to adoption, particularly technology. Managerial principles, such as organizational structure, governance, well-defined workflows, and adherence to regulation and policy play large roles in technology acceptance by end-users, customers, and patients.

Drawing from the Technology Acceptance Model (TAM), which describes how user acceptance affects patients and clinicians in the journey toward abandoning traditional care methods for new technology and innovative approaches. Two of the key drivers of technology acceptance within the TAM framework include the following:

- How the innovative method or technology is diffused into the organization
- How the environment is configured to support the use of the technology

Both drivers of TAM require defined governance and management support to be successful. Additional operational factors such as clinical workflow, regulation, technical workflows, security, and financial workflow will play important roles in the decision to purchase, implement, and adopt a technology.

According to Molfenter et al., existing technology adoption research has discovered that many factors can affect decisions to adopt and continue to use a technology. At the individual level, the TAM describes how user acceptance affects patients' and clinicians' willingness to abandon traditional practices in favor of new technologies [14–16]. Beyond the individual level, explanatory models of organizational decisions to adopt a technology have emerged based on two prominent frameworks: diffusion of innovations and the technology-organization-environment framework [17]. These models describe the fundamental role of management support and how factors such as clinical workflow, regulatory policy prohibiting and facilitating use, concerns regarding information security, and financial/reimbursement policy toward the technology affect the decision to purchase, implement, and use a technology [35].

The role of leadership and their support and practice innovation in technology adoption will also play a major role in laying the foundation for success. Teamwork and cooperation of line-level staff and program management will further drive the adoption of certain technologies. It will be vital to continue to activate these roles as future research on interventions in technology adoption are explored and implemented [35].

Conclusion

Telehealth finance and successful telehealth business models are sources of insight to a metamorphosis continuing to demonstrate value to the respective stakeholders of telehealth. The design and vision for an excellent telehealth business model is not a fortuitous product, but rather a creative organization of key financial variables and governance with a focus on delivering high quality patient care through technology. The chapter authors recommend any leader designated with accountability or responsibility for telehealth needs to understand and recognize the distinguishing value these programs produce. Telehealth leaders have the exciting and noble duty to be transparent and deepen the knowledge, best practices, and information available to grow and mature telehealth well into the future, further informing future discussions and considerations on telehealth business models and financial details.

References

1. Pereira F. Business models for telehealth in the US: analyses and insights [Internet]. Smart Homecare Technology and TeleHealth. 2017 [cited 2019 Mar 7]. Available from: https://www.dovepress.com/business-models-for-telehealth-in-the-us-analyses-and-insights-peer-reviewed-fulltext-article-SHTT.
2. Lighter D. Advanced performance improvement in health care: principles and methods. Sudbury: Jones & Bartlett Learning; 2009. 461 p.
3. Ozcan YA. Analytics and decision support in health care operations management. Hoboken: Wiley; 2017. 814 p.
4. Arkwright B, Jones J, Osborne T, Glorioso G, Russo J. View of Telehealth governance: an essential tool to empower today's healthcare leaders. [cited 2018 Jul 23]. Available from: https://telehealthandmedicinetoday.com/index.php/journal/article/view/12/5.
5. Saunders CL, Brennan JA. Achieving high reliability with people, processes, and technology. Front Health Serv Manag. 2017 Summer;33(4):16–25.
6. Lunney M, Lee R, Tang K, Wiebe N, Bello AK, Thomas C, et al. Impact of telehealth interventions on processes and quality of care for patients with ESRD. Am J Kidney Dis [Internet].

2018 Apr 23 [cited 2018 May 21];72(4):592–600. Available from: https://www.ajkd.org/article/S0272-6386(18)30547-X/abstract.
7. Kulcsar M, Gilchrist S, George MG. Improving stroke outcomes in rural areas through telestroke programs: an examination of barriers, facilitators, and state policies. Telemed J E Health. 2014;20(1):3–10.
8. Mechanic OJ, Kimball AB. Telehealth systems. In: StatPearls [Internet]. Treasure Island: StatPearls Publishing; 2018 [cited 2018 Jul 13]. Available from: http://www.ncbi.nlm.nih.gov/books/NBK459384/.
9. Lacktman N. Medicare payments for telehealth increased 28% in 2016: what you should know [Internet]. [cited 2018 Jul 13]. Available from: http://www.foley.com/medicare-payments-for-telehealth-increased-28-in-2016-what-you-should-know-08-28-2017/.
10. Lacktman N. OIG report: CMS paid practitioners for telehealth services that did not meet Medicare requirements [Internet]. Health Care Law Today. 2018 [cited 2018 May 21]. Available from: https://www.healthcarelawtoday.com/2018/04/16/oig-report-cms-paid-practitioners-for-telehealth-services-that-did-not-meet-medicare-requirements/.
11. Office of Inspector Gen. CMS paid practitioners for telehealth services that did not meet Medicare requirements audit (A-05-16-00058) 04-05-2018 [Internet]. [cited 2018 Jul 13]. Available from: https://oig.hhs.gov/oas/reports/region5/51600058.asp.
12. Office for Civil Rights. Notification of enforcement discretion for telehealth remote communications during the COVID-19 nationwide public health emergency. 2020. Available from: https://www.hhs.gov/hipaa/for-professionals/special-topics/emergency-preparedness/notification-enforcement-discretion-telehealth/index.html.
13. Edgerton SS. A pilot study investigating employee utilization of corporate telehealth services. Perspect Health Inf Manag [Internet]. 2017 Oct 1 [cited 2018 May 21];14(Fall):1g. Available from: https://www.ncbi.nlm.nih.gov/pmc/articles/PMC5653955/.
14. Binder W, Cook J, Gramze N, Airhart S. Telemedicine in the intensive care unit: improved access to care at what cost? Crit Care Nurs Clin North Am. 2018;30(2):289–96.
15. Chen J, Sun D, Yang W, Liu M, Zhang S, Peng J, et al. Clinical and economic outcomes of telemedicine programs in the intensive care unit: a systematic review and meta-analysis. J Intensive Care Med. 2018;33(7):383–93.
16. Plazzotta F, Sommer JA, Marquez Fosser SN, Luna DR. Asynchronous dermatology teleconsultations using a personal health record. Stud Health Technol Inform. 2018;247:690–4.
17. Rat C, Hild S, Serandour J, Gaultier A, Quereux G, Dreno B, et al. Use of smartphones for early detection of melanoma: systematic review. J Med Internet Res [Internet]. 2018 [cited 2018 May 21];20(4):e135. Available from: http://www.jmir.org/2018/4/e135/.
18. Flaten HK, St Claire C, Schlager E, Dunnick CA, Dellavalle RP. Growth of mobile applications in dermatology – 2017 update. Dermatol Online J [Internet]. 2018 Jan 1 [cited 2018 May 21];24(2):13030. Available from: https://escholarship-org.proxy.lib.ohio-state.edu/uc/item/3hs7n9z6.
19. Charlston S, Siller G. Teledermatologist expert skin advice: a unique model of care for managing skin disorders and adverse drug reactions in hepatitis C patients. Aust J Dermatol. 2018;59(4):315–7. https://doi.org/10.1111/ajd.12803. Epub 2018 Mar 23.
20. Center for Connected Health Policy. Telehealth policy barriers. 2016.
21. Duff-Brown B. Measuring return on investment in health care [Internet]. 2016 [cited 2020 July 1]. Available from: https://healthpolicy.fsi.stanford.edu/news/global-health-economics-consortium-tackles-complex-issue-societal-returns-health-care.
22. Medicare Learning Network. Telehealth services. 2018.
23. Leslie M, Virani R. Realizing value with Telehealth in Chronic Condition Management (CCM) programs. Poster presented at 2016.
24. Skibinski D. Beware the telemedicine Trojan Horse – MedCity News [Internet]. [cited 2018 Jul 13]. Available from: https://medcitynews.com/2017/09/beware-telemedicine-trojan-horse/.

25. Eramo L. How to measure ROI of telemedicine: an Oklahoma health system shares some insights – MedCity News [Internet]. 2017 [cited 2018 May 21]. Available from: https://medcitynews.com/2017/04/how-to-measure-roi-of-telemedicine/?rf=1.
26. Qubty W, Patniyot I, Gelfand A. Telemedicine in a pediatric headache clinic. Neurology [Internet]. 2018 [cited 2018 May 21];90(19):e1702–e1705. Available from: http://n.neurology.org/content/90/19/e1702.long; Brohman M, Green M, Dixon J, et al. Community paramedicine remote patient monitoring (CPRPM): benefits evaluation & lessons learned 2015/17. 2018 Apr.
27. Berman SJ, Wada C, Minatodani D, Halliday T, Miyamoto R, Lindo J, et al. Home-based preventative care in high-risk dialysis patients: a pilot study. Telemed J E Health. 2011;17(4):283–7.
28. Announcing Next Gen ACO Results, CMS Administrator Verma Makes the Case for Moving ACOs to Two-Sided Risk [Internet]. Healthcare Innovation. [cited 2019 Mar 7]. Available from: https://www.hcinnovationgroup.com/policy-value-based-care/article/13030646/ announcing-next-gen-aco-results-cms-administrator-verma-makes-the-case-for-moving-acos-to-twosided-risk; Medicare Program; Medicare Shared Savings Program; Accountable Care Organizations-Pathways to Success [Internet]. Federal Register. 2018 [cited 2019 Mar 7]. Available from: https://www.federalregister.gov/documents/2018/08/17/2018-17101/medicare-program-medicare-shared-savings-program-accountable-care-organizations-pathways-to-success.
29. Bortniker AF, Geilfuss CF II. "Pathways to success:" CMS publishes final rule modifying the Medicare shared savings program [Internet]. Health Care Law Today. 2019 [cited 2019 Mar 7]. Available from: https://www.healthcarelawtoday.com/2019/01/07/pathways-to-success-cms-publishes-final-rule-modifying-the-medicare-shared-savings-program/.
30. Medicare Program; Medicare Shared Savings Program; Accountable Care Organizations-Pathways to Success and Extreme and Uncontrollable Circumstances Policies for Performance Year 2017 [Internet]. Federal Register. 2018 [cited 2019 Mar 7]. Available from: https://www.federalregister.gov/documents/2018/12/31/2018-27981/medicare-program-medicare-shared-savings-program-accountable-care-organizations-pathways-to-success.
31. How Henry Ford Physician Network made the numbers work in the Next Generation ACO [Internet]. Healthcare Finance News. [cited 2019 Mar 7]. Available from: https://www.healthcarefinancenews.com/news/how-henry-ford-physician-network-made-numbers-work-next-generation-aco.
32. Center for Connected Health Policy. Telehealth cost effective/efficient studies/pilots/programs [Internet]. 2013. Available from: https://www.cchpca.org.
33. Walsh T, Goerlich C. You're probably measuring telehealth ROI wrong. Use these 6 metrics to do it right [Internet]. 2017 [cited 2018 Jul 13]. Available from: http://www.advisory.com/ research/market-innovation-center/the-growth-channel/2017/05/telehealth-roi.
34. A Guide for Telemedicine Service Vendor Contracting: Applying Traditional Contracting Considerations in a New Arena [Internet]. [cited 2019 Feb 18]. Available from: https://www.bakerdonelson.com/a-guide-for-telemedicine-service-vendor-contracting-applying-traditional-contracting-considerations-in-a-new-arena.
35. Molfenter T, Brown R, O'Neill A, Kopetsky E, Toy A. Use of telemedicine in addiction treatment: current practices and organizational implementation characteristics. Int J Telemed Appl [Internet]. 2018 Mar 11 [cited 2018 May 21];2018:3932643. Available from: https://www.ncbi.nlm.nih.gov/pmc/articles/PMC5866865/.

Chapter 4
Telehealth Development, Implementation, and Sustainability Challenges: An Introduction into the Telehealth Service Implementation Model (TSIM™)

Shawn R. Valenta, Meghan Glanville, and Emily Sederstrom

Introduction

According to Liezl van Dyk in "A Review of Telehealth Service Implementation Frameworks," there are many complex factors (see Table 4.1) that can impact the success of developing and implementing telehealth services [1]. In that article, van Dyk describes how the success rate of telehealth services has been disappointing and a holistic implementation approach is needed. In this chapter, we review some of the early frameworks that van Dyk researched and how they apply to current telehealth challenges. In addition, we provide specific examples throughout the lifecycle of a telehealth service that highlights those complex factors that can impact the development and implementation of a telehealth service. Finally, we conclude with a brief introduction into the Telehealth Service Implementation Model (TSIM™), which was developed and matured out of the Medical University of South Carolina, one of only two HRSA-designated National Telehealth Centers of Excellence in the United States. TSIM is a guiding framework that was created to support the efficient and effective development, implementation, and long-term sustainability of high quality telehealth services.

Table 4.1 Factors impacting the success of telehealth services

Technology	Organizational structures	Change management	Economic feasibility	Legislation
Societal impacts	Perceptions	User-friendliness	Evaluation and evidence	Policy and governance

S. R. Valenta (✉)
Medical University of South Carolina, Johns Island, SC, USA
e-mail: valentas@musc.edu

M. Glanville
MUSC Center for Telehealth, Medical University of South Carolina, Charleston, SC, USA

E. Sederstrom
Department of Strategic Planning, OU Medicine, Oklahoma City, OK, USA

© Springer Nature Switzerland AG 2021
D. W. Ford, S. R. Valenta (eds.), *Telemedicine*, Respiratory Medicine,
https://doi.org/10.1007/978-3-030-64050-7_4

Barriers to the Diffusion of Telehealth

Since telehealth introduces a form of healthcare innovation into the traditional care delivery system, it is impacted by similar factors that can be a barrier to the adoption of any new innovation or technology. Grigsby et al. first assessed the diffusion of telemedicine and the challenges of predicting a rate of adoption considering the many complex and dynamic factors impacting that process [2]. Tanriverdi and Iacono identified the following four key barrier categories for the diffusion of implementing telehealth services: (1) technical barriers, (2) behavioral barriers, (3) economical barriers, and (4) organizational barriers [3].

While technical barriers continue to decline with the increased adoption and knowledge of technology overall, there are still substantial hurdles to implementing a new telehealth technology platform or device. New technology often brings a level of anxiety or fear with the process of attempting something new, both for the providers and the patients. This hesitancy should not be underestimated, but instead, it should be accounted for and addressed with adoption processes and procedures. Healthcare organizations need to ensure that there are processes in place to properly educate, train, and support healthcare providers and patients with telehealth technology.

Behavioral barriers to telehealth adoption can be significant as many people are hesitant to change. The integration of telehealth services into the traditional clinical workflow can be extremely disruptive, and early development and implementation challenges and resistance to change are to be expected, requiring effective change management to overcome those challenges. The following four key components have been associated with effective change management: (1) change leadership, (2) employee (team) engagement, (3) communication, and (4) employee (team) commitment [4]. Telehealth champions have been determined to be crucial in executing successful change leadership by helping to promote the telehealth service, legitimize the initiative, and build relationships with key stakeholders along the way [5]. In addition, establishing a systematic way to develop and implement telehealth services with clear roles and responsibilities will improve team and provider engagement, ultimately increasing the likelihood of creating a successful telehealth service.

Economical barriers can be both internal and external to an organization. Examples of internal economical barriers may include limited funding (i.e., budget) for telehealth initiatives and poor understanding or execution of effective telehealth business models. Establishing a governance structure with sophisticated financial planning and management will help optimize the budget and create sustainable telehealth services. The most significant external economical barrier is the limited and variable telehealth reimbursement policies across the country. While telehealth policies continue to improve overall, reimbursement is often cited as a major barrier to telehealth adoption [6]. As telehealth policies continue to evolve, the telehealth services must adapt with those changes. It is imperative to have strong billing compliance expertise involved in the telehealth service development process. As telehealth reimbursement rules mature, organizations should have a process to review those changes and adapt the telehealth services to optimize revenue collections.

Organizational barriers are rooted in the challenges of integrating telehealth services into the traditional organizational structure and existing clinical workflows. Organizations often struggle with scaling telehealth pilots into successful, sustainable services, because telehealth services are often developed as siloed initiatives outside of the existing system [1]. Organizations need to establish formalized processes and provide institutional support to integrate telehealth services into their existing healthcare system. By having a systematic way to plan, prioritize, develop, implement, and promote telehealth services, organizations will be able to navigate many of the complex factors that have historically challenged the integration of telehealth services into the traditional healthcare system.

Seven Core Principles for the Successful Development of Telemedicine Services

Yellowlees emphasized that effective change management was at the core of successfully developing telehealth services and that the costs, both financial and psychological, of failing to implement a telehealth service properly could have a significant long-term negative impact on a healthcare organization [7]. He notes that very little telehealth advancement occurred in the 1980s, potentially due to many of the failures that occurred with telehealth projects of the 1960s and 1970s. Yellowlees said that the most significant lesson learned when implementing a telehealth service is that it must be integrated into the existing healthcare environment. He identified the following seven core principles as likely to improve the chances of developing successful telehealth services: (1) telemedicine applications and sites should be selected pragmatically, rather than philosophically, (2) clinician drivers and telemedicine users must own the systems, (3) telemedicine management and support should follow best-practice business principles, (4) the technology should be as user-friendly as possible, (5) telemedicine users must be well trained and supported, both technically and professionally, (6) telemedicine applications should be evaluated and sustained in a clinically appropriate and user-friendly manner, and (7) information about the development of telemedicine must be shared. When applying these core principles to the current practice of developing and implementing telehealth services, some common themes are present.

- Principle 1: Telemedicine applications and sites should be selected pragmatically, rather than philosophically

Sometimes telehealth service ideas come from healthcare executives without clinician involvement, and this can lead to a project being initiated without a physician champion identified and/or provider capacity available to deliver the service. Telehealth initiatives need "champions" to navigate the many complex factors and change management challenges of integrating a telehealth service into the traditional system. In addition, telehealth services should be created based on current demand. While a gap analysis may show data that a particular area has a "need" for a clinical service, unless the local healthcare providers or patients demonstrate a "demand," that telehealth service will likely suffer from low utilization. Finally, the telehealth service should address a problem of increasing access, improving quality, and/or reducing costs. Telehealth services should not be implemented if the problem they are intended to solve cannot be articulated.

- Principle 2: Clinician drivers and telemedicine users must own the systems

This principle really focuses on the importance of the physician champions and their involvement in selecting the technologies that they, and their colleagues, will use to transform the way they deliver care. Technology should be selected objectively and be led by the needs of the clinical service. This is a key component of the change management process and one that is often overlooked by many organizations. The users must feel comfortable with the technology and have a level of buy-in to help navigate any early implementation challenges.

- Principle 3: Telemedicine management and support should follow best-practice business principles

Yellowlees warned of putting the responsibility of telehealth implementations on "project teams" that lack both clinical and practical telehealth experience. Some organizations place themselves at risk of this if they run their telehealth teams out of their information technology (IT) departments and too much focus is placed on the technology. Telehealth is not an IT project; it is the implementation of a new clinical service. Between the two, there is a significant difference in skillset required for a successful development and implementation process. Many organizations have found success by centralizing their telehealth support teams and standardizing their processes, but a strong clinical strategy and physician champions should be at the core of those telehealth teams.

- Principle 4: The technology should be as user-friendly as possible

Some of the early challenges with telehealth technology was that the solutions were often big and bulky, expensive, and difficult to use. As technology continues to evolve, the telehealth solutions on the market are transitioning to be more computer-based systems that are easier to use and less expensive. In order to achieve full adoption of telehealth, the technology must be user-friendly and integrate seamlessly into a clinician's workflow. If the use of the technology becomes a burden on the clinician's workflow and clinical efficiency, utilization will suffer, and the telehealth service will eventually fail.

- Principle 5: Telemedicine users must be well trained and supported, both technically and professionally

Yellowlees recommended that if a telehealth team was to have one motto it should be "Train, train and train again." He placed a lot of focus on getting providers used to the technology in non-clinical activities, such as meetings and educational sessions. As telehealth has continued to advance and technology has become more prevalent, the most vital component of training is on executing the workflow effectively. As telehealth has become more integrated into the traditional delivery system, the training on the workflow is not only specific to the provider. Supporting departments, such as an admit transfer center receiving a call for a time-sensitive telestroke consultation, and supporting personnel (e.g., tele-presenter) must also be trained and demonstrate proficiency of their roles and responsibilities. In addition, training on appropriate telehealth documentation and billing is important to stay compliant with state and federal regulations and maximize reimbursement opportunities. Organizations need a systematic way to train providers prior to go-live, review the process to assess competency, and provide ongoing support to make adjustments and improvements along the way as the service continues to evolve.

- Principle 6: Telemedicine applications should be evaluated and sustained in a clinically appropriate and user-friendly manner

In an ever-changing reimbursement system that continues to shift toward value-based payments, organizations need to understand successful telehealth business models and be able to evaluate the value of their investments. In order to be able to successfully sustain telehealth services, outcome metrics should be established to continually evaluate financial and operational performance. Identifying key performance metrics will assist organizations with improving telehealth service delivery to ensure they are meeting the needs of all relative parties, including assessing their own value on investment.

- Principle 7: Information about the development of telemedicine must be shared

Yellowlees stressed the importance of deeper research on telehealth services. While telehealth research has definitely evolved over the last couple of decades, well-designed, high quality scientific research is still limited in the field of telehealth. Telehealth has been proven to show a high satisfaction by a majority of patients [8], but more health economic research needs to be conducted to examine the cost-effectiveness of new delivery models. While some delivery models such as telestroke have demonstrated cost-savings [9], other modes of telehealth, such as direct-to-consumer telehealth for acute respiratory infections, may increase utilization and healthcare costs [10]. More information and research on telehealth must be shared to improve the overall cost-effective and high quality delivery of care.

Five Factors Influencing Service Integration

Finch et al. completed a longitudinal qualitative study that assessed 12 teledermatology services and identified the following five factors that supported the successful integration of those services: (1) policy context, (2) perceived benefit and related commitment, (3) evidence gathering to prove safety and manage risk, (4) reorganizing services, and (5) issues surrounding professional roles and boundary crossing [11]. These five themes and relative factors were identified as either promoting or impeding successful integration of the teledermatology services into the traditional health system.

The context of policy continues to be one of the most relevant factors to tele-health adoption. In the United States, the variability and gaps in telehealth reimbursement policies have made it significantly challenging to create sustainable business models and accelerate adoption of new telehealth technologies and services. In addition, individual state medical boards have often placed restrictions on which medical providers can deliver telehealth services. Until there is more of a national push to simplify payment and licensure issues, many organizations will continue to be slow to adopt telehealth services.

The concept of "perceived benefit and related commitment" can still be a barrier to telehealth integration if the relative stakeholders cannot clearly articulate why the service is being implemented. "What problem does this telehealth solution solve?" should be the first question asked during the planning process when a clear strategy for the telehealth service is being crafted. The service is doomed for failure if that question cannot be answered, but that is not sufficient enough. The answer to that question must be communicated effectively to support successful change management.

In order for large-scale telehealth adoption to occur, processes to support safe, evidence-based care must be matured and risk must be accounted for and managed. The teledermatology services that were successfully sustained were ones that accounted for potential risks and built safeguards into the system to address those issues. An example of this concept can be highlighted when reviewing virtual urgent care, or "direct-to-consumer," services. Concerns have been expressed that direct-to-consumer telehealth visits may pose a risk of increasing the use of antibiotics in children [12]. When risks to safety or quality are identified, it is imperative to account for and act to mitigate or eliminate that risk. For antibiotic usage in direct-to-consumer services, this can be accomplished through formalized quality review processes to assess antibiotic stewardship and adherence to clinical guidelines.

The concept of reorganizing services emphasized that users of telehealth services needed to make continual modifications in order for the service to be successful. A key part of that is understanding the current clinical workflow that the telehealth service is bound to disrupt. Organizations often spend too much time focusing on the technology and not nearly enough time on the process. Organizations need to establish a systematic way to design the new telehealth service, to train and support providers, to assess for ongoing competency with the process, and to continuously identify and execute on process improvement opportunities.

The introduction of telehealth services can also impact the traditional role of different healthcare professionals. In the case of the teledermatology services, there were concerns about an attempt to push too much responsibility toward primary care, but those that demonstrated more flexibility with the process were able to implement successful services. Since telehealth is expected to disrupt the current system, ideally, organizations will capitalize on that opportunity and get different healthcare providers practicing at the top of their license. To realize that potential, policies must be in place to support this transformation. Telehealth has the opportunity to efficiently connect numerous healthcare providers along the care continuum compared to the traditional delivery system.

Advancing Telehealth Service Development and Delivery

Telehealth is experiencing exponential growth, and while resources such as implementation checklists are available to guide early-stage adoption, comprehensive and practical resources to develop and manage telehealth services from the initial idea to sustainable operations are limited. The Telehealth Service Implementation Model or TSIM™ was created to address this need and formalize a guiding framework to support the efficient and effective development, implementation, and long-term sustainability of high quality telehealth services [13]. TSIM was originally implemented at the Medical University of South Carolina (MUSC) in order to enable an institutional goal of comprehensive, enterprise-wide telehealth integration, but the model can serve as a clear guide to any organization attempting to navigate the many complexities of telehealth service development and delivery.

The MUSC Center for Telehealth (Center) was established in 2013 and built upon an 8-year legacy of providing telehealth services that addressed health disparities, initially maternal fetal health, and stroke care, across South Carolina (SC). The founding of the Center was catalyzed by a SC legislative mandate and funding to develop telehealth infrastructure and services that would increase access to care and reduce health disparities. This legislative charge led to the rapid development and expansion of telehealth at MUSC, culminating in over 80 unique telehealth services being offered at over 300 clinical sites across the state within 6 years. Annual telehealth interactions increased from 15,315 to over 308,000 during this time period with 78% of MUSC's services delivered to fully or partially medically underserved SC counties. During this rapid growth phase, the Center experienced meaningful successes and encountered numerous challenges, which have all contributed to the development of the Telehealth Service Implementation Model or TSIM.

There are many challenges and complexities to telehealth service development and, as highlighted by van Dyk, no existing holistic framework to address these. Inspired by van Dyk and the success of established frameworks (e.g., ITIL® for IT service management [14]), MUSC sought to develop a novel framework specifically for successful telehealth implementation. TSIM includes six phases: (1) Pipeline, (2) Strategy, (3) Development, (4) Implementation, (5) Operations, and (6) Continual Quality Improvement. Each phase has associated tasks that must be completed before a service advances to the next phase.

The TSIM framework establishes a holistic approach to incorporating all of the factors that can impact telehealth success, and it provides a common terminology to improve communication between team members. In addition, TSIM allows for a systematic approach to service development, implementation, and service management. The Pipeline phase serves as the entry portal for new telehealth ideas. The Strategy phase ensures that the scope of the telehealth service is clearly defined, and the Development phase is when the service is built, accounting for key steps that must be reviewed and addressed and key stakeholders that must be engaged. In the Implementation phase, providers are trained on the workflow and technology, mock calls are completed, and the operational and technical teams support the go-live process. In Operations, the focus shifts to delivering high quality, reliable telehealth services that continue to improve the patient and provider experience. Continual Quality Improvement occurs throughout the framework, identifying and optimizing process, people, and platform problems.

Ultimately, TSIM enables teams to proactively recognize program strengths, weaknesses, and gaps in service development, implementation, and delivery. TSIM has contributed to MUSC becoming nationally recognized for its extensive breadth and depth in telehealth program development, implementation, and evaluation, and in 2017, MUSC was formally designated by the Health Resources and Services Administration (HRSA) as a National Telehealth Center of Excellence.

Conclusion

Telehealth service development is extremely challenging when attempting to integrate telehealth services into the existing healthcare system. There are many complex factors that have to be considered and numerous stakeholders that must be engaged throughout the process. Historical challenges have impeded adoption, which can have a significant negative impact on telehealth investments. However, success is achievable, and a guiding implementation framework, such as TSIM, can be a major catalyst to telehealth adoption and success at any organization.

References

1. Van Dyk LA. Review of telehealth service implementation frameworks. Int J Environ Res Public Health. 2014;11:1279–98.
2. Grigsby J, Rigby M, Hiemstra A, House M, Olsson S, Whitten P. Telemedicine/telehealth: an international perspective. The diffusion of telemedicine. Telemed J E Health. 2002;8:79–94.
3. Tanriverdi H, Iacono CS. Knowledge barriers to diffusion of telemedicine. In: Proceedings of the international conference of the association for information systems, Helsinki, Finland, 14–16 August 1998. p. 39–50.
4. Makumbe W. Predictors of effective change management: a literature review. Afr J Bus Manag. 2016;10(23):585–93.
5. Wade J, Eliott J. The role of the champion in telehealth service development: a qualitative analysis. J Telemed Telecare. 2012;18(8):490–2.
6. Kruse CS, Karem P, Shifflett K, Vegi L, Ravi K, Brooks M. Evaluating barriers to adopting telemedicine worldwide: a systematic review. J Telemed Telecare. 2018;24(1):4–12.
7. Yellowlees PM. Successfully developing a telemedicine system. J Telemed Telecare. 2005;11(7):331–5.
8. Polinski JM, Barker T, Gagliano N, Sussman A, Brennan TA, Shrank WH. Patients' satisfaction with and preference for telehealth visits. J Gen Intern Med. 2016;31(3):269–75.
9. Switzer JA, Demaerschalk BM, Xie J, Fan L, Villa KF, Wu EQ. Cost-effectiveness of hub-and-spoke telestroke networks for ischemic stroke from the hospitals' perspectives. Circ Cardiovasc Qual Outcomes. 2013;6(1):18–26.

10. Ashwood JS, Mehrotra A, Cowling D, Uscher-Pines L. Direct-to-consumer telehealth may increase access to care but does not decrease spending. Health Aff. 2017;36(3):485–91.
11. Finch TL, Mair FS, May CR. Teledermatology in the UK: lessons in service innovation. Br J Dermatol. 2006;156(3):521–7.
12. Ray KN, Shi Z, Gidengil CA, Poon SJ, Uscher-Pines L, Mehrotra A. Antibiotic prescribing during pediatric direct-to-consumer telemedicine visits. Pediatrics. 2019;143(5):e20182491.
13. MUSC (forthcoming). The Telehealth Service Implementation Model (TSIM): a comprehensive guide to telehealth implementation (9780117092129). TSO, London.
14. Axelos. ITIL-IT service management. Axelos Global Best Practice; 2019. https://www.axelos.com/best-practice-solutions/itil. ITIL® is a (registered) Trade Mark of AXELOS Limited. All rights reserved.

Chapter 5
Telehealth Technology, Information, and Data System Considerations

Ragan DuBose-Morris, Michael Caputo, and Michael Haschker

Introduction

In this chapter, concepts exploring the use of telehealth technology to support the provision of pulmonary, critical care, allergy, and sleep medicine clinical services will be presented. Topics include technology and data system considerations, a framework for understanding telehealth technologies, the application of health informatic principles, and future state technology needs. Finally, we pose some concluding thoughts related to these evolving systems of care.

For over 40 years, technology has been woven into critical care patient applications through a range of telehealth processes and equipment including early references to the use of microwave technology to access cardiac auscultation [1]. The evaluation and monitoring of patients has continued to evolve into all areas of critical care and pulmonary specialty services prompting even higher levels of provider engagement [2]. The technology supporting this progress continues to advance in usability and interoperability while demonstrating cost-effective, life-saving outcomes that are effective across care settings [3–5].

While progress has been made in the development of these innovations, additional work remains in the implementation, refinement, and integration of telehealth technologies that ensure safe and reliable healthcare. As systems realize the goal of interoperability, they are faced with increasing pressures to maintain privacy and

R. DuBose-Morris (✉)
Academic Affairs Faculty, Center for Telehealth, Medical University of South Carolina, Charleston, SC, USA
e-mail: duboser@musc.edu

M. Caputo
Department of Information Technology, Marist College, Poughkeepsie, NY, USA

M. Haschker
Telehealth Technologies, Department of Information Solutions, Medical University of South Carolina, Charleston, SC, USA

© Springer Nature Switzerland AG 2021
D. W. Ford, S. R. Valenta (eds.), *Telemedicine*, Respiratory Medicine,
https://doi.org/10.1007/978-3-030-64050-7_5

security protocols across clinical interactions. Intentionally deployed telehealth technologies can help to bridge the care divide while ensuring that clinical, education, and research processes fully support the future state of care.

Technology and Data System Considerations

Telehealth technologies are defined by the American Telemedicine Association as "the remote delivery of health care services and clinical information using telecommunications technology" [6]. This includes a range of services delivered in real-time such a video consults (synchronous), regardless of aligned time such as store-and-forward images or text-based clinical triage (asynchronous), and through numerous devices, app, and informatic exchanges (remote and m-health). In addition to direct clinical consultative services historically defined as telemedicine, "tele" has evolved to include education and research components seeking to address broader health considerations. Hence, the widely accepted use of the term "telehealth."

Specific to telehealth services provided for patients who are most critical or in need of continuous support, there are three main categories of technology application in this domain supported by information and communication technologies (ICT) [7, 8]:

- "Telemonitoring: the use of ICT to monitor patients at a distance"
- "Teleassistance: the provision of clinical care at a distance using ICT"
- "Telerehabilitation: the use of ICT to provide clinical rehabilitation services at a distance" [7]

Examples of these platforms can be seen in numerous use cases that illustrate clinician led innovation (Table 5.1) [7, 9–12].

These processes are made possible by the convergence of information and communication technologies including Bluetooth connectivity, broadband connectivity, electronic health records, standards-based telehealth platforms, health analytics and data warehousing, emerging artificial intelligence (AI) systems, and state/regional health information exchanges. The ability to support the transfer of audio, video, and data is highly dependent on high-speed, high-reliability networks that facilitate the exchange of information using secure and managed systems. Ideally, healthcare systems utilize Open Access Network technologies that serve as the backbone for shared infrastructure [13]. These essential networks make it simpler to develop new services and manage ongoing daily operations through centrally managed, broadband super highways that connect hospitals, clinics, and community endpoints.

For direct-to-patient consultations, mobile applications and remote patient monitoring, adequate cellular and broadband network connections need to be in place [14]. Through the use of more advanced telehealth technology networks, a combination of devices, such as carts, laptops, and cell phones, can be connected through health information management systems and EHR portals for an integrated

Table 5.1 Telehealth application examples by category [7, 9–12]

Category	Application	Technologies	Examples
Synchronous, provider-to-provider	Tele-ICU: continuous patient monitoring systems integrating EHR and analytic systems with highly trained ICU staff	Video/audio communication Telemetry EHR exchange/portal Robotic carts Electronic messaging	Remote monitoring of patients in an ICU by a centrally housed tele-ICU team in a dedicated operations center in partnership with local ICU providers
Synchronous, provider-to-provider or –patient	Tele-consults: urgent or ambulatory specialty consultations conducted using videoconferencing technologies	Videoconferencing applications supported through hardware (e.g., cart) and/or software applications Peripheral devices (e.g., stethoscope)	Connecting providers to providers or to patients for diagnosis, treatment, and/or follow-up consults
Asynchronous, provider-to-patient	m-Health apps: tracking of patient data through device or user input to support follow-up, care coordination, and medication titration	Remote patient monitoring devices (e.g., blood glucose, weight, O_2 sat) Mobile device apps Device dashboards	Monitoring of patients at home for chronic disease management; manage biometrics and provide education

experience that helps to achieve meaningful use mandates [15]. These telehealth connections are made possible by shared investments in technologies, systems, and process that allow for a spectrum of clinical services to be provided for patients as they move through the healthcare continuum – regardless of patient setting.

Investments in Technology

While upfront investments in technology are often some of the largest expenses associated with telehealth programs, improved funding, reimbursement, and contractual revenue sources are streamlining the process of working with vendors to craft solutions for flexibility and scalability. Identifying program goals, resources, and the current state of the technical landscape are essential before initiating investment commitments. Several guides and reports have been generated that help to list steps and resources required for the implementation of a successful program [16]. Given the breadth and changing landscape of technology available for a critical care, pulmonology, allergy, and sleep medicine applications, seeking out technical experts and other telehealth champions who have implemented similar programs and identified best practices is often helpful in the acceleration of the acquisition process.

Basic environmental scans that document information on the current network and hardware conditions for all program endpoints should be completed to reduce redundancy and ensure compatibility. Examples of the site survey categories to include are listed below and should be informed by clinical, administrative, and technical partners, as appropriate:

- Types of network connectivity (wired Ethernet or Wireless 802.11 N signal or better) and available bandwidth as a function of other IT activities
- Signal strength and range of wireless signals and required equipment frequencies (2.4/5 GHz frequencies)
- Dedicated data circuits in each room so wired equipment is portable
- Requirements for public or private IP (Internet Protocol) addressing for devices (informs monitoring)
- Ability to address security and permission issues through firewall port configuration
- Adequate lighting, sound insulation, and storage options for devices
- Onsite/contracted technical support personnel

Telehealth Design Process

As discussed in Chap. 4, utilizing a service development framework that integrates clinical workflows and health information and technology service principles is essential. Such a framework is especially helpful in determining the current state of health information technology and workforce processes required. The use of a service development framework for telehealth is relatively new, but the need for its structure couples with the possibilities of new clinical services through a validated and iterative process [17]. Based on the established strategy for the service, telehealth technologies are designed, operationalized, and managed through a three-stage process. These include the assessment of the recommended equipment and site configurations that will be involved in the provision of clinical services, the vendor selection process, and the installation of a complete system based on parameters established during the initial strategy. Upon completion of the development phase, technologies then transition into go live and operational phases. This phased approach allows for non-technical, clinical experts to determine feasibility and put in place sustainable processes that include ongoing continuous quality improvement initiatives.

Understanding the current state of network infrastructure, hardware and software applications, and mobile/monitoring device capabilities allows telehealth teams to develop programs that are scalable and sustainable. Table 5.2 provides examples of technologies in the past, present, and future clinical domains [18–21].

The existing technologies and services related to these telehealth domains are relatively ubiquitous, affordable, and user-friendly, but they are also continually evolving. Multiple studies have shown the efficacy as well as potential additional use cases of these technologies when embedded across clinical domains [2, 22–25]. More importantly, they demonstrate that in many cases, small interventions can have significant impacts for patients. Still, the evolving nature of the services,

Table 5.2 Origin, current state, and projections for future state development of telehealth technology [18–21]

Domains	Origin products	Current state products	Future state (research and development)
Tele-ICU	Closed, in-facility networks used for continuous remote monitoring	Continuous monitoring of spoke ICUs by central tele-ICU operations center Telemetry with artificial intelligence or algorithmic capabilities EHR access and/or EHR exchanges Carts/robotic video units In-room emergency buttons	Greater integration of artificial intelligence into regional and national networks of ICUs Improving integration of EHR systems and exchanges to reduce technical barriers Development of real-time lab systems Virtual reality modeling
Asthma care	Video specialty consults for follow-up using primary care or school-based clinics as originating sites	Electronic stethoscopes and cameras (peripheral devices) Remote peak flow monitoring Pulse oximeters Remote inhaler monitoring devices Medication adherence monitoring through sensor technology and mHealth	Equipping patients/families with remote monitoring devices and apps that feed into portals with real-time trend information Improving care coordination and patient education through apps
Sleep medicine	Video specialty consults for diagnosis via primary care clinics or home-based connections	Physiological monitoring Management of positive airway pressure (PAP) equipment	Refined PAP devices Integrated systems with real-time, device monitoring Ongoing clinical and education services through app portals (text and video features) Predictive analytics through AI

coupled with the limited evidence for individual devices, limits readily accessible data for quality assurance testing. Larger scale healthcare systems that have implemented programs can serve as resource labs for the dissemination of outcomes. When properly assessed, quality vendor data can be used in the purchasing and implementation decision-making process [26].

Of increasing importance is the rapid development of digital health, or mHealth, including wearable, implantable, and smart devices. The insertion of these technologies into the telehealth service, education, and research processes are potentially beneficial when usability, reliability, efficacy, and cost-effectiveness results can be provided [12, 18, 27, 28]. Technological processes must also fit into the existing and future clinical workflows for the provider teams responsible for patient medication management and care coordination. Underpinning all of these conversations is the essential requirement that all devices, networks, and applications meet stringent security protocols in order to maintain patient and provider confidentiality, trust, and communication [29].

Telehealth device and solution vendors in the pulmonary, critical care, and sleep domains appear to be relatively limited compared to other video or text-focused service providers. Based on a review of a recent listing of over 250+ telehealth-related vendors, the following 12 met the inclusion criteria for pulmonary, critical care, and/or sleep medicine focused service [30]:

- *Advanced ICU Care (St. Louis)*. Advanced ICU Care is a tele-ICU provider that has implemented and managed tele-ICU programs in partnership with hospitals across the United States.
- *Bernoulli (Milford, Conn.)*. Bernoulli creates software and hardware designed to accelerate the flow of real-time medical device data to providers, which includes patient safety surveillance and virtual ICU solutions.
- *Cloudbreak Health (Columbus, Ohio, and El Segundo, Calif.)*. Cloudbreak Health provides more than 1 million minutes of telemedicine consultation each month, linking patients and providers through the company's telehealth marketplace. The company supports around 75,000 encounters per month at more than 700 hospitals, addressing telepsychiatry, telestroke, tele-ICU, and telesitting functions.
- *Medtronic (Dublin, Ireland)*. Medtronic is focused on medical devices and technology solutions that monitor patients across the care continuum in the hospital and at home.
- *MetTel (New York City)*. MetTel provides telehealth infrastructure for mobile devices, enterprise mobile management, vital sensors, procurement and financing, and support telecommunications.
- *Nokia (Cambridge, Mass.)*. Nokia creates devices to track and improve activity, sleep, weight, heart health, and environmental issues. Some of the devices include wireless blood pressure monitors and Wi-Fi-enabled scales.
- *Nonin Medical (Plymouth, Minn.)*. Nonin Medical focuses on technologies and products, such as pulse and regional oximeters, capnographs, sensors, and software.
- *Oxitone Medical (Kfar Saba, Israel)*. Oxitone Medical developed a bracelet with oxygen saturation, pulse and motion biosensors, as well as a companion patient management app for continuous patient monitoring and transition care services.
- *PeraHealth (Charlotte, N.C.)*. PeraHealth provides real-time, predictive analytics solutions based on data science and clinical care best practices. The solutions are designed to help clinicians identify at-risk patients and tackle initiatives, such as reducing unplanned ICU transfers and readmissions.
- *Sensogram Technologies (Plano, Texas)*. Sensogram Technologies is a research and development company focused on biosensors that allows for continuous remote and mobile monitoring of vital signs.
- *Telehealth Sensors (North Aurora, Ill.)*. Telehealth Sensors works with clients to program monitors for their specific needs, including continuous monitoring capabilities, and focuses on creating inconspicuous products to protect the privacy of users.

- *VeeMed (Sacramento, Calif.)*. VeeMed is a global telemedicine company focused on virtual clinical patient healthcare services and advanced telemedicine technology in chronic care, nephrology, pulmonary medicine, neurology, and mental healthcare.

National Communication Technologies

The broadband networks and backend infrastructures that support the provision of telehealth are essential for quality, reliable connectivity. The need for high-speed data services (>100 Mbps download) to support telehealth technologies has been established by the US Federal Communications Commission [31]. Even with significant investment and the creation of a Health Care Connect Fund that supports a superhighway for healthcare transmissions, many areas of the nation lack adequate broadband connectivity [32]. In addition, identified physician provider shortages, often in rural communities, are generally in parallel with reduced communication connectivity. This combination of both provider and modern communication connectivity shortages exacerbates issues of access, equity, and sustainability. Figures 5.1, 5.2, and 5.3 illustrate the challenges faced from a systemic perspective including technical networks and the intersection of healthcare workforce distribution.

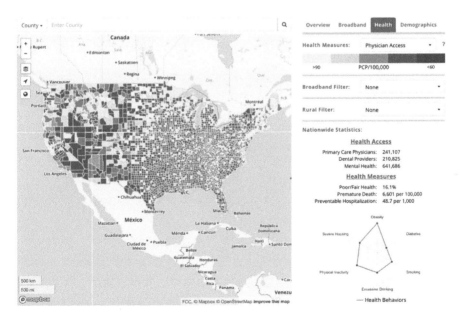

Fig. 5.1 Primary care physicians per 100,000 residents. (From the FCC Mapping Broadband Health in America 2017 Report [33])

Residential Fixed Internet Access Service Connections per 1000 Households by Census Tract
As of June, 2017

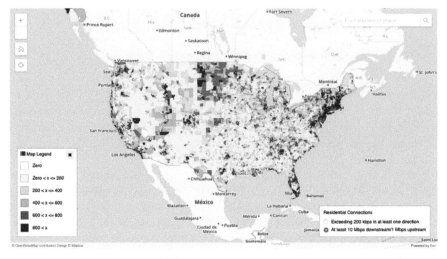

Map shows the number of residential fixed Internet access service connections per 1,000 households based on June 2017 Form 477 broadband subscribership data. Includes data on connections by census tract for both service over 200 kbps in at least one direction and service at least 10 Mbps down / 1 Mbps up. For more information, see the Internet Access Services Reports.

Fig. 5.2 Residential fixed internet access per 100 households by census tract. (From the FCC Report on Residential Fixed Internet Access [34])

LTE Coverage by Number of Providers - YE 2017

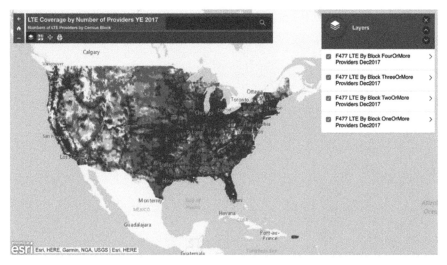

Based on Form 477 Dec. 2017 and 2010 Census data. Note that the number of service providers in a census block represents network coverage only. Network coverage does not necessarily reflect the number of service providers that actively offer service to individuals located in a given area.

Fig. 5.3 2017 LTE coverage number by ISP. (From the FCC F477 LTE by Provider Block [35])

National Communication Infrastructure: Relevance to Telehealth

Adequate Internet connectivity ranks as one of the largest barriers to telehealth implementation. Successful telehealth services require Internet connectivity and bandwidth, which meets the minimum requirements of the telehealth services offered. The use of real-time video coupled with the sharing of medical device peripherals, such as otoscopes and stethoscopes, require Internet access and adequate bandwidth to deliver the telehealth network traffic in real time and without interruption to the telehealth service. In 2017, the Federal Communication Commission undertook an important endeavor to nationally map and link broadband and health data for every county in the United States. The result was a series of interactive maps that allow users insights into the intersections between these pivotal resources. These tools can help inform public and private sector efforts to close gaps in both connectivity and healthcare at the local, state, and national levels. The following sections highlight some of the key findings from the FCC project Mapping Broadband Health in America [33]. Important operational definitions include the following:

- Internet access is defined as the ability of individuals and organizations to connect to the Internet using computer terminals, computers, and other devices; and to access services such as email and the World Wide Web.
- Bandwidth describes the maximum data transfer rate of a network or Internet connection. It measures how much data can be sent over a specific connection in a given amount of time.

Mapping Broadband Health in America 2017 allows users to visualize, overlay, and analyze broadband and health data at the national, state, and county levels. By using the mapping tool as a starting point for looking at the broadband and health sectors, one can see the path to a more connected, healthier country. Areas with sufficient broadband and health offerings have increased access to healthcare resulting in a more connected and healthier population.

While the nation continues to make progress in broadband access, millions of Americans still lack access to adequate broadband, especially in rural areas and on Tribal lands. This baseline map visualizes broadband access at the county level and identifies connectivity gaps – the lighter the county color, the lower the percentage of households with robust broadband access.

Figure 5.1 [33] depicts FCC data related to healthcare provider access by county. Provider types include primary care physicians, dental and mental health providers only. Corresponding with limited broadband access, rural areas have significantly less access to healthcare providers than in most urban areas.

Basic infrastructure support for healthcare, such as that provided through FCC funding, is essential for the adoption and growth of telehealth services. The needs addressed are multifaceted and span all economies of scale including the ability to extend telehealth services to remote locations and into home settings. Fixed Internet service at home with a minimum level of 10 Mbps is far from a universal commodity, as seen in Fig. 5.2 [34].

Figure 5.2 demonstrates the average amount of available bandwidth to connected households in Dec 2017. Rural areas are subject to limited choices for Internet Service Providers (ISPs) and bandwidth offerings from those providers.

Increased access to telehealth services also rely on cellular connectivity. The use of cellular services offer access to larger patient populations and can more easily address connectivity issues in rural areas where running dedicated Internet connections into each household is not feasible. While LTE ("Long Term Evolution," cellular data service) is available across much of the country, there are incomplete areas with service offerings and coverage of up to four carriers demonstrated in Fig. 5.3. The FCC's report does not speak to actual quality, speed, or reliability for those cellular networks [35].

Continued investments in infrastructure, both wired broadband and cellular connectivity, are essential. Even in states that have made significant use of FCC funds and shared resources, connectivity ranks as one of the largest barriers to implementation [36]. Lessons learned include plans for equipment renewals, reinvestment of revenues, and partnering with similar missioned entities, such as research universities, to share solutions.

Brief Overview of Telehealth Technology in the Context of Pulmonary, Critical Care, and Sleep Medicine

The technologies involved in tele-ICU services are numerous and include utilizing videoconferencing codecs, physiological monitoring, electronic health records and exchanges, monitoring platforms, desktop computers, telehealth carts, robotic devices, and, in some cases, patient devices such as smart phones and tablets. These technologies are provided, monitored, maintained, and contractually facilitated by large healthcare systems, often in partnership with established industry partners. Information technology support is available 24/7 through help desk and remote monitoring systems. Due to the complex nature of these systems, the provider-side workforce is required to be highly proficient in multiple technology systems, able to conduct higher-level troubleshooting, and adaptable to different staffing shift and payment models. Combined, the benefits derived from these technologies are highly dependent upon human variables and the creative application of multiple systems across existing domains (Fig. 5.4).

For more consultative telehealth applications (Fig. 5.5), such as pediatric asthma management, the nature of the clinical interaction is supported through more user-friendly and cost-effective applications. While the initial diagnosis may have been made through an in-person consult, the administration of medication through a school-based clinic by a school nurse is a common example of utilizing clinical personnel in nontraditional settings to improve the health of populations through telehealth. Patient education on the need for medications, the administration of inhaled medication, care coordination to ensure medication compliance, and

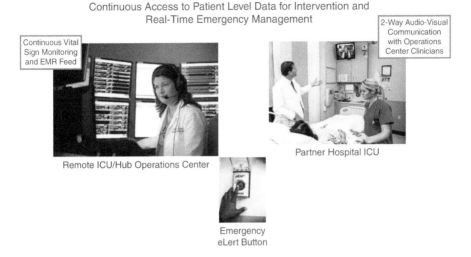

Continuous Access to Patient Level Data for Intervention and Real-Time Emergency Management

Continuous Vital Sign Monitoring and EMR Feed

2-Way Audio-Visual Communication with Operations Center Clinicians

Remote ICU/Hub Operations Center

Partner Hospital ICU

Emergency eLert Button

Fig. 5.4 Visualization of tele-ICU at hub and spoke sites

Fig. 5.5 School-based telehealth and asthma management

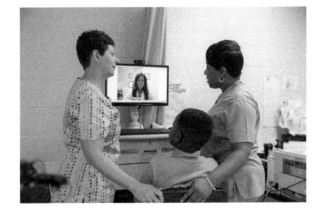

ongoing consultation with specialty providers ensure that patients remain in the community where they are currently located and receive more frequent, lower cost, and high quality care [37, 38].

Additional tele-consultative models have also been effective in urgent and emergent settings to support pediatric intensive care unit patients using telehealth modalities to assess patients in rural and community hospitals for decisions related to triage, condition acuity, need for transportation (air or ground), and additional clinical assessment. These interventions have resulted in improved outcomes for patients within the originating hospital location and upon transfer, if needed, to an academic medical center setting [39]. More importantly, from a technology perspective, existing services have been applied to support these consults. This includes the use of carts and video codecs to transmit information from a community setting while utilizing existing desktop or laptop technologies within a clinic or home-based environment (Fig. 5.5). Having one additional level of visual data coming from the video codec, allows for providers to reduce uncertainty and their tendency to error on the side of caution in patient transports to tertiary medical centers. Follow-up and next-day assessments utilizing the same technologies help ensure providers and patients remain assured that the patient is receiving care in the optimal location.

Traditionally, the initial sleep medicine assessment conducted with a patient in an overnight lab has been the primary way in which the diagnosis of sleep-related disorders has occurred. Being able to bring equivalent levels of technology for physiological assessments and monitoring, video observation and audio feedback into the home setting, changes how the science behind the assessment can be conducted [18, 40, 41]. As shown in Fig. 5.6, the application of telehealth technology outside the traditional sleep medicine clinic setting improves the use of prescribed devices such as the CPAP (Continuous Positive Airway Pressure) machine, the ability to review nocturnal biometric inputs through sensors, and the ability of patients to provide more immediate feedback on the effectiveness of their treatment plan [12]. This allows for the adjustment or maintenance of medication, equipment, and/or other therapies. Exciting examples of technology that can be worn, ingested, and positioned in proximity of the patient have transformed the type of real-world readings that are available through dashboard technology for both patients and their providers.

With the development of mobile apps and additional biometric sensors, the next phase of progress is to empower patients to better understand their own sleep status, record metrics throughout the day that might impact overnight readings and make adjustments to their lifestyles based on the data. Here, the advances in technology will come in partnership with health apps and processes developed for a more general public use case. Applications already on the market that help with the treatment of mental health disorders, smoking cessation, and the lack of movement, buttress

Fig. 5.6 Example of telehealth sleep medicine process. (From McNeil [56])

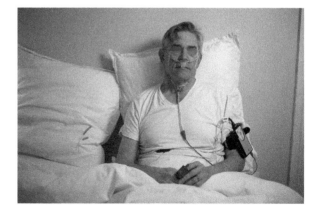

into the ecosystem of tools that can be deployed for patients needing additional monitoring and support [42].

Data Systems and Integrations

From the earliest recorded uses of data systems to transmit electronic records related to a patient's medical history, more complex systems such as tele-ICUs benefit from the ability to support real-time and higher-level critical decision-making through interoperability and secure networking. Health information exchanges have accelerated the development of information sharing between providers, institutions, and systems [43]. Current operational guidelines for telehealth services such as a tele-ICU, acute specialty care consults, and the monitoring of patients remotely within home-based networks call for the deliberate and dutiful integration of health informatics and data analytics when possible [9, 40]. This is one of the areas of the largest opportunities and equal challenges due to the complex and crucial nature of the processes being interwoven. Being awash in a proverbial sea of remote patient monitoring metrics or having numerous warning indicators alerting a provider to varying degrees of clinical concern further complicates the provision of these types of telehealth services. Too much information can be no information at all. In addition to integrated solutions that simplify the decision-making process while highlighting important clinical indicators, interoperability can assist to mitigate possible adverse reactions based on the integration of higher order analytics and AI.

The required telecommunications support making these network functions also dictate that services are built with shared understanding for protocols that ensure patient privacy and support high reliability [23]. Each device, network port, and software interface must support secure transmissions and data storage solutions. As more systems shift toward cloud-based platforms for data storage, transmission, and analysis, telehealth administrators should remain vigilant that these processes are properly maintained across all sites supporting the provision of care.

Using data to inform decision-making processes should be an iterative cycle that technology can better inform. By focusing on the expectations of how providers will receive patient data and patients will receive provider input, each end of the healthcare continuum, can be better supported [44]. Tele-ICUs cannot function without high levels of interoperability and most often serve as their own health information exchanges. Emergent and urgent teleconsultation that immediately impact transport and care decisions for patients through specially consultation also rely upon integrated systems that support data transmission across geographic and institutional barriers. Without systems that can take individual data points gathered from sensors, video and audio input, and patient-reported metrics, the potential of these remote sleep medicine services will not be fully realized [41].

With this foundation of knowledge related to information and communication systems, the conversation moves into the area of the technology needed to fully support new models of population health and achieving the triple aim of improved healthcare, cost, and outcomes. Programs seeking to utilize telehealth should determine the simplest and most appropriate level of technological interventions to support patients and their families in home and community settings. Technologies can be used to prevent community members from experiencing significant health events through improved lifestyle initiatives, self-monitoring of health conditions and education initiatives appropriate for multiple age, health literacy, and socioeconomic audiences. Expensive and complicated systems are not always operational or sustainable outside pilot studies. Being able to serve patients using the appropriate level of technologic support has been shown to have the largest impact on patient outcomes [12].

Data-Driven Research Methodologies for Telehealth Technology

Research methodologies, including qualitative and quantitative assessments, provide a clearer understanding of quality outcomes [3, 4, 45, 46]. Studies looking specifically at the human factors such as usability and effectiveness have shown that significant design challenges remain [47]. Known issues include being able to quickly identify areas for technology troubleshooting, addressing integration issues across platforms, establishing reliability metrics that are scalable, and reducing barriers to adoption due to poor user interfaces and workflows that are not optimized for established clinical monitoring needs. Further and ongoing research is needed during the procurement and implementation phases to ensure HIPAA compliance in established clinical settings and in-home settings outside the traditional consideration of most health informatic processes [48].

For all systems, programs need to conduct comparisons of applications, devices, and process for ease of use by multiple parties including clinicians, providers, and technical personnel tasked with supporting the services [48]. Utilizing a variety of data analysis methods to understand not only how the technology is being implemented, but also what outputs are measurable is essential from the beginning of any program design [9]. In addition, qualitative research methodologies and analyses need to be implemented in order to validate the technology continuum, assess usability and patient satisfaction components associated with technology, as well as better understand the needs for training, research, and care coordination [8, 44, 45, 47, 49]. Better understanding the "how and why" related to the provision of telehealth services can help to inform the iterative technology development process as seen in Fig. 5.7.

Moving from a position of utilizing established, secure telehealth technologies and processes toward a validated state based on integrated data and feedback inputs provides programs with ways to ensure current state functionality while achieving

Fig. 5.7 Telehealth
technology evaluation
process: from security to
validity

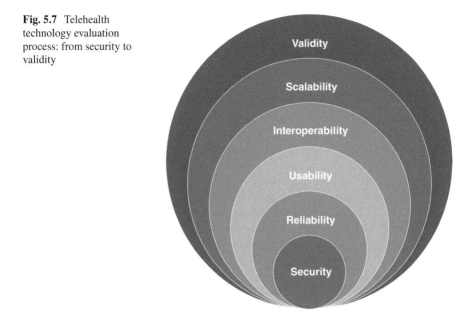

future state sustainability. Highly validated processes also afford programs with the ability to layer additional programs without having to invest in surplus equipment, portals, applications, processes, or even human resources. Strong foundational support that creates interoperable programs allows for the transcendence of historic IT service models. This also helps with cost containment and utilizing shared investments to obtain quantity pricing for short-term equipment purchases with flexibility to scale up for larger system purchases as more sites and services come onboard.

Additional Considerations for Implementing Telehealth Technology

Current technology barriers include the continued need to utilize systems and products that have not been tested to scale. Given the large technological investments that precede the development of most telehealth services, having significant initial investment and sustainability plans is essential. Understanding an organization's most complex, as well as simplest, unmet telehealth technology need is important. The use of pilot testing to ensure that technology and system purchases meet load testing protocols is recommended. Technologies can be crowd-sourced from a funding model perspective (federal, state, local, private donor, and reinvestment of revenues), so it is important to make sure that all stakeholders benefit from the initial investment as well as understand their roles and responsibilities for helping to make the program a success. The technology is only one element of organizational innovation and partnership. Due diligence is required to make sure that all vendor products are vetted not only internally, but ideally also via soliciting experiences with comparable healthcare systems who have implemented the proposed solution previously.

Several federal and state statutes apply to the purchase of telehealth equipment for the use of healthcare systems. Resources are available through the Center for Connected Health Policy website (https://www.cchpca.org) that address HIT-specific implications for telehealth as well as additional considerations for broadband usage and access as stipulated in Net Neutrality legislation [50].

Developing a template for robust inventory control as well as tracking systems upfront will help with legal and compliance questions. This will also ensure that adequate technical support can be provided through equipment inventory documentation. In addition, evolving knowledge bases can be invaluable when dealing with complex and interwoven systems that span multiple software versions and hardware designs. Being able to address life-cycle and upgrade issues, as well as budgeting for yearly recurring cost, will be essential for long-term success.

Developing a multilayered and audience-specific training education program is essential for supporting the technology needs of telehealth programs. Not only do providers need specific and timely information regarding the devices and services that they will be using to provide care, they also need ongoing education to ensure continual quality improvement processes are being effective. Formal training programs are the natural evolving result of any telehealth service that moves into full-scale operations. Partners with resources at academic health centers, institutions of higher education, and community health educators can be enlisted to ensure that the training is appropriate from a health and technology literacy perspective.

Emphasis on Multi-Level and Interprofessional Training

To ensure that future generations of providers are prepared to integrate telehealth into their clinical practices, telehealth programs should consider enlisting support from and taking advantage of curriculum opportunities within formal and informal programs of study for the undergraduate and graduate health professions schools [51]. Trainees not only can help to bring great ideas and energy to the technology development table, they can also help accelerate telehealth growth via higher rates of provider knowledge and engagement [52]. Formal training guidelines as well as board certification documentation may become required in the future. In addition, masters and doctorate-level health information technology professionals offer a wealth of specialized expertise that can accelerate program development and help mitigate inevitable technical issues through the design of integrated systems and that are supported through interprofessional operations.

Applying Telehealth Technology Considerations to Professional Society Position Statements

Several professional associations have already begun to draft formal position statements regarding telehealth, and these can be helpful in providing guidance for the prioritization of service development and implementation activities. The Taskforce on Telemedicine in Allergy [22] supports the following position statements in Table 5.3. In reviewing these guidelines from a technology perspective, the authors

Table 5.3 Taskforce on telemedicine in allergy position statements

Taskforce on telemedicine in allergy position statements	% Technology dependent
Telemedicine is a method of healthcare delivery that may enhance patient-physician collaborations and adherence, reduce overall medical cost, improve health outcomes, and increase access to care.	Moderate
Telemedicine activities should account for varying literacy and technologic literacy levels and strive for ease of use in interface design, content, and language.	High
The use of telemedicine must be secure and compliant with state and federal regulations.	High
Healthcare practices should confirm that medical liability coverage includes a provision for telemedicine services.	Low
Clinical judgment should be used when determining the scope and extent of telemedicine services provided to patients.	High
Quality assurance measures should be in place to track patient satisfaction, physician performance, and clinical outcomes whether at an originating site or via home-based telemedicine care.	Moderate
Live interactive video visits with allergy patients should be at the same standard of care and held to the same standards of professionalism and ethics as in-person consultations.	Low
Live interactive video visits should be reimbursed at the same rate as in-person care, and there should be transparency and understanding of payer reimbursement for different modes of telemedicine delivery.	Low
Best practices for safety in telemedicine care delivery should be followed at all times.	High
Roles, expectations, and responsibilities of practitioners involved in the delivery of allergy care should be clearly defined.	Low
Appropriate technical standards should be upheld throughout the telemedicine care delivery process and specifically meet the standards set forth by HIPPA.	High*
Time for data management, quality processes, and other aspects of care delivery related to telemedicine encounters should be accounted for by the organization and recognized in value-based care delivery models.	Moderate
Telemedicine use for allergy care is likely to expand with broader telehealth applications in medicine; further research into effect and outcomes is needed.	Low
A streamlined process for multistate licensure would improve access to specialty care while allowing states to retain individual licensing and regulatory authority.	Low

perceive low-moderate-high dependences for the degree to which technology is a factor. The highest dependency is noted (*).

Considerations, Recommendations, and Conclusions

The creation of various telehealth models to support pulmonary, critical care, and sleep medicine stems from the clinical necessity and growing focus on population health models. This chapter has provided a foundation for knowledge specific to telehealth technology and data system considerations specific to these domains. As part of this foundation, there is a reference framework that outlines current and future state telehealth technologies, discusses the application of health informatic principles, and sets the stage for next-generation technology integration.

Areas of continued and future research specific to telehealth technologies center on usability testing, clinical integration processes, and consumer-led implementations. Several healthcare innovations on the horizon include the use of more robust 5G cellular networks and the evolution of the "Medical Internet of Things (IoT)" [53]; virtual payment and date exchanges, such as blockchain [54]; and advances in biomedical sensors to extend care into telerehabilitation settings [55]. Usability testing, clinical and research outcomes validated through randomized clinical trials and multi-year cost analysis directly related to the use of telehealth technologies remain areas for continued exploration. Providers and patients alike are charged with investigating ways that they can empower the health of communities through small-scale innovations and large-scale advancement supported by integrations using telehealth technologies.

References

1. Murphy RLH, Block P, Bird KT, Yurchak P. Accuracy of cardiac auscultation by microwave. Chest [Internet]. 1973 Apr 1 [cited 2019 Feb 23];63(4):578–81. Available from: https://www.sciencedirect.com/science/article/pii/S0012369215478389.
2. Avdalovic MV, Marcin JP. When will telemedicine appear in the ICU? J Intensive Care Med [Internet]. 2019 Apr [cited 2019 Feb 3];34(4):271–6. Available from: http://journals.sagepub.com/doi/10.1177/0885066618775956.
3. Armaignac DL, Rubens M, Williams L-MS, Gidel LT, Veledar E, Saxena A, et al. Impact of telemedicine on mortality, length of stay, and cost among patients in progressive care units. Crit Care Med [Internet]. 2018 May [cited 2019 Feb 3];46(5):728–35. Available from: http://www.ncbi.nlm.nih.gov/pubmed/29384782.
4. Vranas KC, Slatore CG, Kerlin MP. Telemedicine coverage of intensive care units: a narrative review. Ann Am Thorac Soc [Internet]. 2018 Nov 1 [cited 2019 Feb 3];15(11):1256–64. Available from: https://www.atsjournals.org/doi/10.1513/AnnalsATS.201804-225CME.
5. Liu M, Chen J, Zhang S, Yang W, Ren C, Peng J, et al. Clinical and economic outcomes of telemedicine programs in the intensive care unit: a systematic review and meta-analysis. J

Intensive Care Med [Internet]. 2017 Jul 22 [cited 2019 Feb 24];33(7):383–93. Available from: http://journals.sagepub.com/doi/10.1177/0885066617726942.
6. American Telemedicine Association. Telehealth FAQs – ATA Main [Internet]. 2018 [cited 2019 Feb 24]. Available from: http://www.americantelemed.org/main/about/about-telemedicine/telemedicine-faqs.
7. Hassan E. Tele-ICU and patient safety considerations. Crit Care Nurs Q [Internet]. 2018 [cited 2019 Feb 24];41(1):47–59. Available from: http://insights.ovid.com/crossref?an=00002727-201801000-00006.
8. Kairy D, Lehoux P, Vincent C, Visintin M. A systematic review of clinical outcomes, clinical process, healthcare utilization and costs associated with telerehabilitation. Disabil Rehabil [Internet]. Taylor & Francis. 2009 [cited 2019 Feb 24];31:427–47. Available from: http://www.tandfonline.com/doi/full/10.1080/09638280802062553.
9. Davis TM, Barden C, Dean S, Gavish A, Goliash I, Goran S, Graley A, Herr P, Jackson W, Loo E, Marcin JP, et al. Guidelines for TeleICU operations. Telemed J E Health. 2016;22(12):971–80.
10. Gurbeta L, Badnjevic A, Maksimovic M, Omanovic-Miklicanin E, Sejdic E. A telehealth system for automated diagnosis of asthma and chronical obstructive pulmonary disease. J Am Med Inform Assoc [Internet]. 2018 Sep 1 [cited 2019 Feb 3];25(9):1213–7. Available from: https://academic.oup.com/jamia/article/25/9/1213/4999662.
11. Raza T, Joshi M, Schapira RM, Agha Z. Pulmonary telemedicine: a model to access the sub-specialist services in underserved rural areas. Int J Med Inform [Internet]. 2009 Jan 1 [cited 2019 Feb 3];78(1):53–9. Available from: https://www.sciencedirect.com/science/article/pii/S1386505608001287.
12. Hilbert J, Yaggi HK. Patient-centered care in obstructive sleep apnea: a vision for the future. Sleep Med Rev [Internet]. 2018 Feb 1 [cited 2019 Feb 3];37:138–47. Available from: https://www.sciencedirect.com/science/article/pii/S1087079217300448.
13. Hmida HA. Open access network (OAN) and fixed mobile convergence (FMC): foundation for a competitive new business model. Adv Sci Lett [Internet]. 2018 Nov 1 [cited 2019 Feb 24];24(11):8651–9. Available from: http://www.ingentaconnect.com/content/10.1166/asl.2018.12318.
14. Musselwhite C, Freeman S, Marston HR. An introduction to the potential for mobile eHealth revolution to impact on hard to reach, marginalised and excluded groups. Cham: Springer; 2017 [cited 2019 Mar 4]. p. 3–13. Available from: http://link.springer.com/10.1007/978-3-319-60672-9_1.
15. Doarn CR, Pruitt S, Jacobs J, Harris Y, Bott DM, Riley W, et al. Federal efforts to define and advance telehealth – a work in progress. Telemed J E Health [Internet]. 2014 May [cited 2019 Feb 3];20(5):409–18. Available from: http://www.ncbi.nlm.nih.gov/pubmed/24502793.
16. Force AA of SMTIT. Sleep telemedicine implementation guide [Internet]. Darien; 2017. Available from: https://j2vjt3dnbra3ps7ll1clb4q2-wpengine.netdna-ssl.com/wp-content/uploads/2018/06/SleepTelemedicineImplementationGuide.pdf.
17. Sadegh SS, Khakshour Saadat P, Sepehri MM, Assadi V. A framework for m-health service development and success evaluation. Int J Med Inform [Internet]. 2018 Apr 1 [cited 2019 Feb 24];112:123–30. Available from: https://www.sciencedirect.com/science/article/pii/S1386505618300030.
18. Singh J, Badr MS, Diebert W, Epstein L, Hwang D, Karres V, et al. American Academy of Sleep Medicine (AASM) position paper for the use of telemedicine for the diagnosis and treatment of sleep disorders. J Clin Sleep Med [Internet]. 2015 Oct 15 [cited 2019 Feb 3];11(10):1187–98. Available from: http://jcsm.aasm.org/ViewAbstract.aspx?pid=30218.
19. Bruyneel M. Technical developments and clinical use of telemedicine in sleep medicine. J Clin Med [Internet]. 2016 Dec 13 [cited 2019 Feb 3];5(12):116. Available from: http://www.ncbi.nlm.nih.gov/pubmed/27983582.
20. Krainin J. Is the sleep lab obsolete? Telehealth and the future of sleep medicine [Internet]. [cited 2019 Mar 1]. Available from: https://accountable-care.healthcaretechoutlook.com/cxoinsights/is-the-sleep-lab-obsolete-telehealth-and-the-future-of-sleep-medicine-nid-273.html.

21. Zundel KM. Telemedicine: history, applications, and impact on librarianship. Bull Med Libr Assoc [Internet]. 1996 Jan [cited 2019 Feb 24];84(1):71–9. Available from: http://www.ncbi.nlm.nih.gov/pubmed/8938332.

22. Elliott T, Shih J, Dinakar C, Portnoy J, Fineman S. American College of Allergy, Asthma & Immunology position paper on the use of telemedicine for allergists. Ann Allergy Asthma Immunol [Internet]. 2017 Dec 1 [cited 2019 Mar 1];119(6):512–7. Available from: http://www.ncbi.nlm.nih.gov/pubmed/29103799.

23. Kahn JM, Le TQ, Barnato AE, Hravnak M, Kuza CC, Pike F, et al. ICU telemedicine and critical care mortality: a national effectiveness study. Med Care [Internet]. 2016 Mar [cited 2018 Sep 14];54(3):319–25. Available from: http://www.ncbi.nlm.nih.gov/pubmed/26765148.

24. Yoo B-K, Kim M, Hoch JS, Sasaki T, Marcin JP. Selected use of telemedicine in intensive care units based on severity of illness improves cost-effectiveness. Telemed J E Health [Internet]. 2017 Jan 1 [cited 2019 Feb 3];24(1):21–36. Available from: https://www.liebertpub.com/doi/10.1089/tmj.2017.0069.

25. Ambrosino N, Fracchia C. The role of tele-medicine in patients with respiratory diseases. Expert Rev Respir Med [Internet]. Taylor & Francis. 2017 [cited 2019 Feb 3];11(11):893–900. Available from: https://www.tandfonline.com/doi/full/10.1080/17476348.2017.1383898.

26. Wider J. Tips for giving your organization a telehealth checkup. Health Manag Technol [Internet]. 2017;38(4):6–9. Available from: http://search.ebscohost.com/login.aspx?direct=true&db=cin20&AN=122290022&site=ehost-live.

27. Inskip JA, Lauscher HN, Li LC, Dumont GA, Garde A, Ho K, et al. Patient and health care professional perspectives on using telehealth to deliver pulmonary rehabilitation. Chron Respir Dis [Internet]. 2018 [cited 2018 Sep 14];15(1):71–80. Available from: https://open.library.ubc.ca/cIRcle/collections/facultyresearchandpublications/52383/items/1.0368693.

28. Ambrosino N, Vagheggini G, Mazzoleni S, Vitacca M. Telemedicine in chronic obstructive pulmonary disease. Breathe [Internet]. 2016 Dec [cited 2018 Sep 14];12(4):350–6. Available from: http://www.ncbi.nlm.nih.gov/pubmed/28210321.

29. U.S. Department of Health and Human Services. HITECH Act Enforcement Interim Final Rule | HHS.gov [Internet]. Special Topics. 2015 [cited 2019 Feb 3]. Available from: https://www.hhs.gov/hipaa/for-professionals/special-topics/hitech-act-enforcement-interim-final-rule/index.html.

30. Dyrda L. 250+ telehealth companies to know | 2018 [Internet]. Becker's Hospital Review. 2018 [cited 2019 Mar 2]. Available from: https://www.beckershospitalreview.com/lists/250-telehealth-companies-to-know-2018.html.

31. Federal Communications Commission. Connecting America: The National Broadband Plan. BalchCom [Internet]. 2010:1–376. Available from: http://download.broadband.gov/plan/national-broadband-plan.pdf.

32. Healthcare Connect Fund – Rural Health Care Program – USAC.org [Internet]. [cited 2019 Mar 2]. Available from: https://www.usac.org/rhc/healthcare-connect/default.aspx.

33. Connect2HealthFCC – Mapping Broadband Health in America 2017 [Internet]. 2017 [cited 2019 Mar 2]. Available from: https://www.fcc.gov/reports-research/maps/connect2health/#ll=34.016242,-97.646484&z=4&t=insights&inb=in_bb_access&inh=in_pcp_access&dmf=none&inc=none&slb=50,100&slh=0,0.0024&zlt=county.

34. Federal Communications Commission. Residential fixed internet access service connections per 1000 households by census tract [Internet]. [cited 2019 Mar 2]. Available from: https://www.fcc.gov/reports-research/maps/residential-fixed-Internet-access-service-connections-per-1000-households-by-census-tract/.

35. LTE Coverage by Number of Providers – YE 2017 [Internet]. FCC F477 LTE by Provider Block. 2018 [cited 2019 Mar 2]. Available from: https://www.fcc.gov/reports-research/maps/lte-coverage-number-providers-ye-2017/.

36. Wildeman MK. SC continues to invest in telehealth, but Internet connections lag. Post & Courier [Internet]. 2019 Mar 3. Available from: https://www.postandcourier.com/business/sc-

continues-to-invest-in-telehealth-but-Internet-connections-lag/article_231c8572-349f-11e9-b4e9-ef122b41ecb2.html.

37. Cormack CL, Garber K, Cristaldi K, Edlund B, Dodds C, McElligott L. Implementing school based telehealth for children with medical complexity. Segal R, editor. J Pediatr Rehabil Med [Internet]. 2016 Sep 2 [cited 2019 Mar 2];9(3):237–40. Available from: http://www.medra.org/servlet/aliasResolver?alias=iospress&doi=10.3233/PRM-160385.

38. Garber KM. School-based telehealth: an effective and innovative way to improve access to care. J Pediatr Health Care [Internet]. 2016 Jul 1 [cited 2019 Mar 2];30(4):306–7. Available from: https://linkinghub.elsevier.com/retrieve/pii/S0891524516300682.

39. Olson CA, McSwain SD, Curfman AL, Chuo J. The current pediatric telehealth landscape. Pediatrics [Internet]. 2018 Feb 27 [cited 2018 Jun 18];141(3):e20172334. Available from: http://www.ncbi.nlm.nih.gov/pubmed/29487164.

40. Zia S, Fields BG. Sleep telemedicine: an emerging field's latest frontier. Chest [Internet]. 2016 Jun 1 [cited 2019 Feb 3];149(6):1556–65. Available from: https://www.sciencedirect.com/science/article/pii/S0012369216416120.

41. Verbraecken J. Telemedicine applications in sleep disordered breathing: thinking out of the box. Sleep Med Clin [Internet]. 2016 Dec 1 [cited 2019 Feb 24];11(4):445–59. Available from: http://www.ncbi.nlm.nih.gov/pubmed/28118869.

42. Fino E, Mazzetti M. Monitoring healthy and disturbed sleep through smartphone applications: a review of experimental evidence. Sleep Breath [Internet]. 2018 Apr 23 [cited 2019 Mar 2];23(1):13–24. Available from: http://link.springer.com/10.1007/s11325-018-1661-3.

43. Braunstein ML. A brief history and overview of health informatics. In: Health informatics on FHIR: how HL7's new API is transforming healthcare [Internet]. Cham: Springer International Publishing; 2018 [cited 2019 Mar 2]. p. 3–12. Available from: http://link.springer.com/10.1007/978-3-319-93414-3_1.

44. Vitacca M, Montini A, Comini L. How will telemedicine change clinical practice in chronic obstructive pulmonary disease?. Ther Adv Respir Dis [Internet]. SAGE Publications. 2018 [cited 2019 Feb 3];12:1753465818754778. Available from: http://www.ncbi.nlm.nih.gov/pubmed/29411700.

45. Lee JT, Kerlin MP. ICU telemedicine and the value of qualitative research for organizational innovation. Am J Respir Crit Care Med [Internet]. 2018 Nov 15;199(8):935–6. Available from: https://www.atsjournals.org/doi/10.1164/rccm.201811-2074ED.

46. Rak KJ, Kahn JM, Hravnak M, Ashcraft LE, Barnato AE, Angus DC, et al. Identifying strategies for effective telemedicine use in intensive care units. Int J Qual Methods [Internet]. 2017 Dec 6 [cited 2019 Mar 1];16(1):160940691773338. Available from: http://journals.sagepub.com/doi/10.1177/1609406917733387.

47. John Doyle D, Dahaba A, LeManach Y. Advances in anesthesia technology are improving patient care, but many challenges remain. BMC Anesthesiol [Internet]. 2018 [cited 2018 Sep 14];18(1):39. Available from: https://doi.org/10.1186/s12871-018-0504-x.

48. Agnisarman SO, Chalil Madathil K, Smith K, Ashok A, Welch B, McElligott JT. Lessons learned from the usability assessment of home-based telemedicine systems. Appl Ergon [Internet]. 2017 Jan 1 [cited 2019 Mar 1];58:424–34. Available from: https://www.sciencedirect.com/science/article/pii/S0003687016301557.

49. Bernocchi P, Scalvini S, Galli T, Paneroni M, Baratti D, Turla O, et al. A multidisciplinary telehealth program in patients with combined chronic obstructive pulmonary disease and chronic heart failure: study protocol for a randomized controlled trial. Trials [Internet]. 2016 Dec 22 [cited 2018 Sep 14];17(1):462. Available from: http://trialsjournal.biomedcentral.com/articles/10.1186/s13063-016-1584-x.

50. Health Information Technology | CCHP Website [Internet]. Center for Connected Health Policy. [cited 2019 Mar 4]. Available from: https://www.cchpca.org/telehealth-policy/health-information-technology.

51. DuBose-Morris R, Cochran K, Epps CC. Applying statewide innovation through infrastructure and partnership. J Natl AHEC Organ. 2013;XXIX(1):28–31.

52. McGowan BA, Henry BW, Block DE, Ciesla JR, Vozenilek JA. Clinician behaviors in telehealth care delivery: a systematic review. Adv Health Sci Educ [Internet]. 2016 Oct 1 [cited 2018 Jun 18];22(4):869–88. Available from: http://link.springer.com/10.1007/s10459-016-9717-2.

53. Magsi H, Sodhro AH, Chachar FA, Abro SAK, Sodhro GH, Pirbhulal S. Evolution of 5G in Internet of medical things. In: 2018 International Conference on Computing, Mathematics and Engineering Technologies (iCoMET) [Internet]. Piscataway: IEEE; 2018 [cited 2019 Mar 5]. p. 1–7. Available from: https://ieeexplore.ieee.org/document/8346428/.

54. Halamka JD, Alterovitz G, Buchanan WJ, Cenaj T, Clauson KA, Dhillon V, et al. Top 10 block-chain predictions for the (near) future of healthcare. Blockchain Healthc Today [Internet]. 2019 Feb 7 [cited 2019 Mar 3]. Available from: https://blockchainhealthcaretoday.com/index.php/journal/article/view/106/108.

55. Cao D, Zhang Z, Liang H, Liu X, She Y, Li Y, et al. Application of a wearable physiological monitoring system in pulmonary respiratory rehabilitation research. In: 2018 11th International Congress on Image and Signal Processing, BioMedical Engineering and Informatics (CISP-BMEI) [Internet]. Piscataway: IEEE; 2018 [cited 2019 Mar 5]. p. 1–6. Available from: https://ieeexplore.ieee.org/document/8633113/.

56. McNeil Jr DG. A sleep apnea test without a night in the hospital. New York Times. 2014. https://well.blogs.nytimes.com/2014/07/21/a-test-you-want-to-sleep-through/.

Chapter 6
People Issues in Telehealth

Katharine Hsu Wibberly and Tina Sweeney Gustin

Introduction

Eight-year-old Emma is yet again at the school nurse' office. She is exhausted, having been up coughing much of the night. She was diagnosed with childhood asthma almost 2 years ago, and since that time her symptoms have gotten progressively worse. Emma lives in a small rural community where there is a part-time nurse practitioner at a rural health clinic and a part-time school nurse who divides her time between four schools in two different counties. Telehealth equipment was recently placed into the school system through grant funding. Unfortunately when the equipment was placed into the schools, training did not take place for the distant providers. Policies were put in place for the school systems, but not the community providers. The school nurse felt that Emma needed to be seen immediately and decided to initiate a telehealth visit with the local nurse practitioner. The school had obtained consents from Emma's parents when the telehealth equipment was placed into the school. The school nurse first confirmed that consent was on file, contacted Emma's mother about her daughter's condition, and initiated the visit with the on-call nurse practitioner. The mother remotely logged on for the visit from her place of employment. Unfortunately at the start of the telehealth visit, the

K. H. Wibberly (✉)
Karen S. Rheuban Center for Telehealth, Mid-Atlantic Telehealth Resource Center, University of Virginia School of Medicine, Charlottesville, VA, USA
e-mail: Kathy.Wibberly@virginia.edu

T. S. Gustin
Center for Telehealth Innovation, Education and Research, College of Health Sciences, Department of Nursing, Old Dominion University, Virginia Beach, VA, USA

© Springer Nature Switzerland AG 2021
D. W. Ford, S. R. Valenta (eds.), *Telemedicine*, Respiratory Medicine,
https://doi.org/10.1007/978-3-030-64050-7_6

nurse practitioner was not located in a quiet office. The nurse practitioner began the appointment while in the grocery store and did not assure the patient and her mother that the appointment was being conducted through a HIPAA secure platform or site location. The nurse practitioner was dressed in casual attire, and seemed to be unaware of how to conduct the virtual visit. Emma's mother was frustrated and asked that the visit stop. She instructed the school nurse that she would pick Emma up and travel the 2 hours to the tertiary hospital for treatment. The school nurse decided to let the school board know that telehealth would not work in this setting and she did not plan to make another consult.

Emma's story is not unique. The specific medical concerns and types of social and environmental factors preventing access to needed care take many shapes and forms. An ever-growing body of evidence supports the use of telehealth when it comes to clinical outcomes, provider support and education, patient and provider satisfaction, and cost-effectiveness. Conversely, there are numerous examples of "failed" telehealth programs such as that described above.

Unquestionably, telehealth is dependent on technology, but the success of a telehealth program is less about the technology and more about the people and workflows that are established. The technology is simply a tool, just as the stethoscope is a tool. Perhaps to better understand issues surrounding the diffusion and adoption of technology, one can glean from the history of the stethoscope:

Today stethoscopes are a typical fixture around doctors' necks …. The practice of percussion and immediate auscultation were popular in physical examinations by the early 1800s. In immediate auscultation, physicians placed their ear directly on the patient to observe internal sounds. A French physician named Rene Laennec (1781–1826) was a firm believer in this method of diagnosis. He worked to refine the auscultation procedure and link the sounds with specific physiological changes in the chest. Immediate auscultation could be an awkward procedure, particularly for female patients. In 1816, Laennec found himself in one of these situations. He rolled a few sheets of thick paper into a tube shape and applied the tube to the woman's chest instead of his ear. Later, he made a more durable instrument out of wood and called it the stethoscope. It was a monaural model that consisted of one tube and was used on one ear. The first practical bi-aural stethoscope was made in 1851 … while many physicians readily adopted monaural stethoscopes, the bi-aural stethoscopes were met with some skepticism. Doctors worried about hearing imbalances caused by using both ears instead of one. For this reason, many doctors continued to use monaural stethoscopes into the early 1900s. [1]

Who would have thought that it would take over 50 years for the stethoscope to become commonplace as a tool in a clinician's practice? The Diffusion of Innovation (DOI) Theory is a theoretical model first developed by Rogers in 1962 that continues to be studied and refined today. DOI is one of the most widely used theories for explaining the process by which an idea or product gains traction over time, ultimately resulting in its adoption. For Rogers [2], "An innovation is an idea, practice, or project that is perceived as new by an individual or other unit of adoption" no matter how long that idea, practice, or project has actually been in existence.

Rogers defined the rate of adoption as "the relative speed with which an innovation is adopted by members of a social system." There are five main factors that influence adoption of an innovation, with relative advantage being the strongest predictor. These five factors include the following:

- *Relative Advantage*: The degree to which an innovation is perceived as being better than the idea it supersedes. Within the context of relative advantage, Rogers also defined two types of innovations: preventive and incremental.

  - A preventive innovation is one that is adopted to decrease the probability of an unwanted future event.
  - Incremental innovations are ones that are perceived to provide a beneficial outcome in a short period of time.
  - Preventive innovations tend to have a slower rate of adoption than incremental innovations.

- *Compatibility*: The degree to which an innovation is perceived as consistent with the existing values, past experiences, and needs of potential adopters.
- *Complexity*: The degree to which an innovation is perceived as relatively difficult to understand and use.
- *Trialability*: The degree to which an innovation may be experimented with on a limited basis. Trialability is positively correlated with the rate of adoption.
- *Observability*: The degree to which the results of an innovation are visible to others.

Rogers posits that innovations offering more relative advantage, compatibility, simplicity, trialability, and observability will be adopted faster than other innovations. Like the stethoscope, adoption of "new" telehealth technologies are constrained by individual beliefs and attitudes, personal and anecdotal experiences, and opportunities for exposure and training. In this chapter, we will take a closer look at three specific "people issues" as they relate to the adoption of telehealth services. These include the following: (1) workforce readiness and engagement; (2) operations and workflow integration; and (3) care model design.

Telehealth Adoption from Perspectives of End-Users

Table 6.1 provides a snapshot of some of the most recent survey findings related to rates of adoption and reasons for adoption or non-adoption. These are placed within the context of four of the five factors described in the DOI Theory outlined above. The "Trialability" factor was omitted, as it was not one that could be ascertained from survey data.

Table 6.1 Adoption of telehealth from end-user perspectives

Target audience	Mid to large employers	Hospitals/providers (inpatient market)	Hospitals/providers (outpatient market)	Patients/consumers
Study	2017 National Business Group (NBG) on Health Survey[a] of 148 large employers (more than 5000 employees) 2017 Willis Towers Watson (WTW) Best Practices in Health Care Employer Survey[b] of 555 mid to large employers (at least 1000 employees)	2017 HIMSS Analytics Survey of Inpatient Telehealth[c] of 136 C-Suite, IT professionals, clinicians, department heads, and HIMSS Analytics LOGIC survey of 5460 US hospitals 2017 Sage Growth Partners (SGP) Survey[d] of over 100 healthcare executives 2018 Deloitte Center for Health Solutions (DCHS) Survey[e] of 624 primary and specialty care physicians	2017 HIMSS Analytics Survey of Outpatient Telehealth[f] of 161 physicians and administrators 2017 Sage Growth Partners (SGP) Survey[d] of over 100 healthcare executives 2018 Deloitte Center for Health Solutions (DCHS) Survey of 624 primary and specialty care physicians	2017 National Business Group (NBG) on Health Survey[g] of 148 large employer 2016 Deloitte Center for Health Solutions (DCHS) Survey of 3,751 adult US Health Care Consumers 2018 Deloitte Center for Health Solutions (DCHS) Survey of US Health Care Consumers
Rate of adoption	96%	71% (HIMSS)	49% of physicians (HIMSS)	20% employees (NBG) 70+% would be willing/ interested in trying it (DCHS2016)
Trends	Adoption of telehealth by large employers has increased sharply since 2014. In 2014, 48% of large employers reported that they had plans to offer telehealth services to employees (NBG)	Adoption of telehealth solutions or services has surged since the study was first conducted. In 2014, it was roughly 54% (HIMSS) After consistently growing 3.5% annually based on study results adoption has increased roughly 9% since 2016 (HIMSS) The most model growth over the last 3 years has been seen in the area of concierge services (eVisits, online consults, and consumer-oriented consults)	While budgets for telehealth today are modest, they are growing. Nearly three-quarters of respondents with existing telehealth solutions expect their telehealth budget to increase next year. These findings demonstrate that adoption rates and budgets for telehealth are on an upswing, but that overall investment is still relatively small (SGP)	While utilization rates are rising, only 20% of employers are currently reporting rates at 8% or higher (NBG)

Relative advantage
The degree to which an innovation is perceived as being better than the idea it supersedes.

Preventive innovation—adopted in order to decrease the probability of an unwanted future event	The continued rise in healthcare costs has made cost management of health benefit programs as the top priority for employers in 2017 and 2018 (WTW)	In the inpatient setting, respondents view telehealth as important for lowering the cost of care (SGP)	In home-based monitoring, respondents see value in lowering the cost of care. However, the value proposition of in-home remote patient monitoring (RPM) is still evolving under value-based reimbursement (SGP)	Consumers want the convenience and are open to technology-aided care, but also need/want assurances from their providers regarding quality of care and protection of patient information (DCHS2016)
Incremental innovations—perceived to provide a beneficial outcome in a short period of time	Employers view telehealth as a way to decrease health system utilization, which in turn will help to contain costs (WTW)	In the inpatient setting, respondents view telehealth as important for alleviating physician shortages and improving access to care, particularly specialty care (SGP) Widespread telehealth adoption has been hindered by the uncertain reimbursement and regulatory landscape. The return on investment for telehealth under fee for service healthcare reimbursement has been challenging (SGP)	Home-based or app-based telehealth is seen as more important for enhancing brand awareness. Executives see potential for telehealth to help them attract and retain patients, and strengthen their brand (SGP) In home-based monitoring, respondents see value in improving outcomes (SGP) Physicians agree that virtual care supports the goal of patient-centeredness. The top three benefits from physicians' perspective are as follows: Improved patient access to care Improved patient satisfaction Staying connected with patients and their caregivers (DCHS2018)	

(continued)

98 K. H. Wibberly and T. S. Gustin

Table 6.1 (continued)

Target audience	Mid to large employers	Hospitals/providers (inpatient market)	Hospitals/providers (outpatient market)	Patients/consumers
Compatibility The degree to which an innovation is perceived as consistent with the existing values, past experiences, and needs of potential adopters	Employers also aim to enhance employee engagement by increasing choice of benefit plans, improving decision support, and offering health wearables and mobile apps (WTW)	Healthcare organizations have invested heavily in electronic medical record systems in the past decade, only to face continued challenges when they try to integrate patient and financial data from disparate sources. They view the integration of a telehealth consult/visit into their workflow as yet one more barrier to efficient care delivery (SGP)	With millennials, being seen at their convenience is more important than building a longitudinal relationship with a physician (SGP) Healthcare organizations increasingly understand telehealth's ability to drive evolving metrics such as consumer satisfaction, brand recognition, and patient acquisition and retention (SGP)	Millennials are more interested in telehealth than any other generation. Millennials report a 20% higher level in interest than seniors. As a whole, seniors have the least interest in using telehealth (DCHS2016) Seniors and consumers who suffer from chronic conditions are less likely to be flexible with the providers they see—41% with a chronic condition and 60% of seniors say they would use telehealth options only with their regular healthcare provider (DCHS2016) The younger the generation, the more flexibility they express regarding their providers: While only 27% of Millennials would limit telehealth to a regular, trusted provider, 33% of Generation Xers and 44% of Baby Boomers would do the same (DCHS2016)

Complexity The degree to which an innovation is perceived as relatively difficult to understand and use	Nearly half of executives estimate that their current telehealth solution fails 15% of the time, yet 70% of executives consider reliable connectivity to be a "must have" (SGP) Healthcare executives want telehealth solutions that are easy to use, easy to navigate, and compatible with their EMRs (SGP)	Tools need to provide an end-to-end experience. For example, if a tool helps patients obtain and track prescriptions but does not allow them to refill medication, many would rather not use that tool at all (DCHS2016)
Observability The degree to which the results of an innovation are visible to others	Emergent use cases such as telestroke have become more mature, to the point that they are widely acknowledged to have transformed the standard of care (SGP)	In our focus groups, once consumers heard personal stories of other group members who had used the technology or were experiencing the chronic condition, more participants were open to trying the technologies

ahttps://www.mobihealthnews.com/content/large-employer-telehealth-adoption-will-hit-96-percent-next-year-survey-says
bhttps://www.willistowerswatson.com/en-US/press/2017/08/us-employers-expect-health-care-costs-to-rise-in-2018
chttps://www.himssanalytics.org/sites/himssanalytics/files/HIMSS%20Analytics%202017%20Inpatient%20Telehealth%20Essentials%20Brief%20Snapshot%20Report.pdf
dSage Growth Partners (February 2018). Defining telehealth's role—the view from the C-suite
ehttps://www2.deloitte.com/insights/us/en/industry/health-care/virtual-health-care-health-consumer-and-physician-surveys.html
fhttps://www.himssanalytics.org/sites/himssanalytics/files/HIMSS%20Analytics%202017%20Outpatient%20Telehealth%20Essentials%20Brief%20Snapshot%20Report_0.pdf
ghttps://www.mobihealthnews.com/content/large-employer-telehealth-adoption-will-hit-96-percent-next-year-survey-says

End-User: Mid to Large Employers

As is apparent from Table 6.1, rates of adoption of telehealth vary significantly based on the type of end-user and seem to correlate relatively well with Rogers' factors. The highest level of adoption was found among mid to large employers. For this group, the "Relative Advantage" was clear. The employers all recognized that traditional cost control techniques alone have not been able to reduce costs. In order to decrease the probability of an unwanted future event (uncontrolled skyrocketing healthcare costs), they looked to telehealth as a preventive innovation. Additionally, these employers also saw telehealth as an incremental innovation. By offering the convenience of telehealth to their employees, they felt that they could rather rapidly decrease health system utilization, which would not only immediately impact healthcare spending, but also decrease time away from work. For this group, innovation is clearly perceived as being better than the ideas that superseded it.

End-User: Hospitals/Providers

Hospitals and inpatient providers had the next highest level of adoption. Telehealth within the inpatient, and particularly the emergent care setting, has had time to come to maturity, to the point where there is "Observability." However, adoption has been hindered by other factors. For example, the "Relative Advantage" is clouded by uncertainties pertaining to reimbursement policies and the evolving shift from volume to value-based care. Many hospitals are still recovering from the implementation of electronic medical records and are skittish about another investment in technology that may or may not enhance care or be easy to use. This impacts both "Compatibility" and "Complexity" in relationship to both perceptions and experiences with technology.

Adoption of telehealth in the outpatient setting, while growing, continues to lag behind the inpatient setting. Within this context, the "Relative Advantage" holds many promises, but the degree to which the innovation is perceived as being better than the in-person in-office care remains unclear.

Provider Issues and Telehealth Adoption

Deloitte [3] offers tactical considerations in four areas for helping physicians/providers adopt virtual care. These include the following:

- Workforce readiness and engagement
- Technology infrastructure and interoperability
- Operations and workflow integration
- Care model design

It should come as no surprise that only one of the four tactical considerations relates to technology. As stated earlier, although there is no doubt that telehealth is dependent on technology, the success of a telehealth program is less about the technology and more about the people and processes that are established. We will therefore take a closer look at these three tactical "people"-related considerations more closely.

Workforce Readiness and Engagement. Despite the adoption of telehealth into various clinical settings, educational programs have lagged behind with the necessary training. Neither medical programs nor nursing programs have been mandated to include didactic content or clinical experiences with telehealth. Curricula are already full and without a mandate from certifying bodies, and most colleges and universities have not elected to introduce telehealth into their programs. Providers are then expected to begin using telehealth technologies with only a brief introduction to the equipment. There are telehealth training programs available for providers interested in additional training. Most of these training programs have a focus on technology, interoperability, reimbursement, HIPAA regulations, and legal and regulatory issues. Some training programs have a focus on programmatic development. Unfortunately most do not address the unique skill set needed to conduct a videoconferencing visit. "Screen side etiquette" is a unique skill set that is not intuitively transitioned from trained bedside etiquette.

Telehealth requires professionals to develop the patient-professional relationship in a different and more deliberate manner [4]. Being an excellent in-person provider does not automatically translate into being a great telehealth provider as this is a different skillset [5]. Providers, regardless of the profession, spend time learning how to demonstrate empathy, provide motivational interviewing, and read body language for in-person visits. They are not, however, trained in methods to translate these skills into a telehealth encounter. Despite the overwhelming use of social media for communication, this type of communication does not translate to telehealth. It has been suggested that this everyday use of technology has lessened individual's abilities to empathize and pick up on non-verbal cues when using technology to communicate [6]. Research has shown that without proper training, even seasoned providers may be unsuccessful in telehealth visits [7]. The best technologies can fail without proper human interaction.

Guidance for Provider Behavior During a Telehealth Interaction

Bulik [7] explored through a mixed-methods study four categories of behavior that should be taught to improve the overall patient-provider relationship with telehealth: (1) verbal categories, (2) non-verbal categories, (3) relational categories, and (4) actions/transactions categories.

Table 6.2 Provider behavior during a telehealth encounter

Behavior categories	Requirements	Check
Provider appearance	Well groomed Clothing choices (limited patterns, avoid dark colors, non-shiny) Limit jewelry	
Distractors	Make sure equipment functioning (check 15-minutes prior) Minimize outside noise Remove clutter from room No eating or drinking Shut door and put a sign on the door regarding the meeting Let others know you will be conducting a telehealth visit Assess lighting—avoid back lighting Limit paper shuffling, pen tapping, etc. Mute microphone when it is not in use Turn pagers and telephones off	
Privacy	Assess the environment for privacy (close door) Assure that there are no other employees in the room Announce who is present on both patient and provider sides Determine if the patient wants to continue with the visit Show the patient the room with the camera Assure patient of equipment security	
Non-verbal communication	Look at the camera and not the patient's face Close-up shots should be used to enhance bonding Minimize charting and looking down Minimize distracting gestures	
Verbal communication	Use purposeful words to display empathy Limit long pauses and dead space Remember pacing of visit Use small talk and conversation	
Empathy	Lean into screen Use words to express empathy Nod Maintain eye contact	

Table 6.2 summarizes some of the human factors and related behaviors that should be considered during a telehealth interaction.

The transmission of a professional appearance is just as important as during an in-person visit. In conjunction to a well-groomed professional appearance when conducting a telehealth encounter, the provider must also consider clothing and jewelry choices. Dark colors and prints should be avoided. Dark colors will wash out the appearance of the presenter, while shapes and patterns may blur on the screen which may distract the receiver [8]. The same is true for jewelry. Glittery bright jewelry may divert attention away from the presenter. Distractors such as outside noise, poorly functioning equipment, clutter in the room, eating, poor lighting, and interruptions from others can be distracting to both the presenter and the receiver [9, 10]. Thus, it is important to close the door prior to a visit, place a sign on the door, and remove all distractors from the desk top and other visual items from behind the presenter. The telehealth presenter must assure that distracting noises such as paper shuffling, tapping pens, and keyboarding is limited. The microphone should be in the mute mode when the presenter is not speaking. At the start of every encounter, the telehealth presenter must first check to assure that both the provider and the patient are in secure private settings. All individuals in each setting should be introduced. If possible, both the provider and the patient should use the telehealth camera to show one another the room. Some states now require that a consent for the telehealth encounter is signed prior to the visit. This should always be checked prior to the encounter [11].

Non-verbal and verbal cues are essential to a successful telehealth encounter. *Non-verbal cues* should first focus on camera placement to assure eye contact when the provider looks at the screen. Close-up shots should be used when possible as this fosters a sense of bonding between the patient and the provider. It is important that the provider purposefully project warmth, interest, and concern to assure a connection with the patient. Ideally, the camera should be mounted on the top of the computer screen and the provider should maintain an eye gaze between the camera and the receiver's image. Looking directly at the receiver's image on screen does not project the appearance of direct eye contact. The provider should ascertain that their image is centered on the screen throughout the visit. If working with a telepresenter, s/he should be mindful of non-verbal behaviors that demonstrate empathy such as leaning in, nodding, and appropriate smiling.

Verbal cues include the introduction of small talk at the start of a telehealth encounter. The telepresenter must maintain congruence between facial and verbal communication, realizing that body language demonstrated during an in-person visit is not seen on a telehealth screen. Silence, while appropriate in an in-person visit, is experienced as awkward long periods of silence during a telehealth encounter. Timing, pacing, and small talk must be purposefully considered.

Empathy is often expressed in-person through touch or body positioning. Other modes of expressing empathy must be deployed during a telehealth visit. Providers can lean into the screen, nod, and assure good eye contact. Each of these methods is a powerful skill in expressing both interest in the patient and empathy. Purposeful word choices of understanding and concern are critical when touch is not an option.

Operations and Workflow Integration

Deloitte [3] states "While workflow may not be the most obvious barrier to adoption, it can be a barrier to usage." Workflow is often understood as the sequence of physical and mental tasks performed by various people within and between work environments. Workflow takes place on multiple levels, and relates to the inter- and intra-organizational relationships that take place between people, both before, during, and after a patient visit. A recent article published in mHealth Intelligence [12] was titled "Telehealth Success Linked to Workflow, Rather than Technology." The opening paragraphs state the following:

> Telehealth is proving its value not because of new technology, but because of better workflows and collaboration.
>
> A program that placed telehealth platforms into 15 primary care clinics at the Los Angeles County Department of Health Services found that wait times for diabetic retinopathy screening were reduced by almost 90 percent—from 158 days to just 17 days. It also greatly improved screening rates for the more than 21,000 patients who were tested between September 2013 and December 2015.
>
> More importantly, researchers said, the project proved that a telehealth platform that splits that workflow between primary care and specialty care providers can achieve greater efficiency and outcomes if done right.

One can expect greater efficiency and outcomes through telehealth when strategic and well-developed workflows are implemented. Lyles and Sarkar [13] discussed the evaluation of the above referenced diabetic retinopathy screening program and stated the following:

> Although these implementation solutions seem straightforward and clear, they actually represent cultural shifts in work responsibilities, as well as expectations on the part of both primary care and specialty professionals and staff … these workflows are multifaceted, given that primary care and specialty care practices often operate with differing training backgrounds, as well as financial incentives, and therefore their ideas of teams must be somewhat reshaped for programs such as this one to succeed. For example, eye clinic professionals (both ophthalmologists and optometrists) need to be convinced that taking in-person DR screening out of their existing workflows—while decreasing the number of nonurgent or benign referrals to their clinic—sufficiently generates enough visits for patients who need higher-level care (possibly including other eye care needs beyond DR). Similarly, primary care professionals need to be educated about the accuracy of telehealth DR screening compared with in-person examinations, and the need to be assured that appropriate monitoring of the quality of the digital images will ensure accuracy for triaging the scarce specialty care resources. In turn, medical assistants and licensed vocational nurses need to feel confident in adding a new task to their day and that they have sufficient training, support, and feedback to maintain quality control.

The success of a telehealth program is predicated on the investment of both time and energy in interpersonal relationships between all affected stakeholders. Engaging, educating, and obtaining buy-in from providers and staff are what will ultimately lead to perceived "Relative Advantage."

Care Model Design. The final tactical human factor consideration is care model design. Whereas operations and workflow are primarily driven by the interactions between healthcare professionals and organizational staff, care model design is driven by the interactions between healthcare professionals and organizational staff with the patient and the patient's family and caregivers. As telehealth becomes more ubiquitous, and the concept of virtual care becomes part of mainstream care delivery, it opens the door to different models of care previously seen as infeasible.

One such model is that of the interprofessional care team. Telehealth is one of the true "team sports." Interprofessional care has several benefits to both the team of healthcare professionals and the patient. This type of care empowers team members, closes communication gaps between professionals and patients, enables more comprehensive patient care, and promotes patient centeredness. As professionals become comfortable with telehelalth and this form of delivery is more readily available, much of this communication and team-based care could be accomplished virtually.

Another care model involves fully engaging family members, friends, and caretakers of the patient. For example, currently in the inpatient setting, a physician will check in with each patient some time during the day, generally in the morning, to see how the patient is doing. These patient rounds may involve a broader care team including nurses, residents, pharmacists, etc. It is in this context that a patient's diagnosis and treatment options are determined. There is unpredictability with regard to the timing of rounds and thus often family who may wish to participate in rounds, are unable to do so. Thus, a number of physicians and hospitals have been implementing "virtual rounds." In some models of virtual rounding, the physician comes into the patient room by way of videoconference, and family members, friends and/or caregivers can be alerted to join by video when the physician arrives. In other models of virtual rounding, the physician physically comes into the patient's room, but enables other members of the care team and family members, friends, and/or caregivers to participate by video. This same concept of the virtual check-in can also take place after the patient is discharged, either to another facility or to home.

Future Directions: Looking Ahead

According to 2016 data from Rock Health [14], 2011 saw just over $1 billion invested in digital healthcare. By 2016, investment levels grew to $4.2 billion and topped $6 billion in 2017. Telehealth is clearly a growth industry, and adoption is forecasted to continue. It is likely that in the future "telehealth" will simply be "healthcare," and telehealth technology will be a typical fixture in every clinician's office in the same way as the stethoscope.

Telehealth will be the engine for enabling patient-centered collaborative care, ultimately bringing to patients the right care, in the right place, at the right time, and with the right team of providers. Team-based care has become a focus of healthcare in the last decade. The Institute of Medicine recommended in 2001 that healthcare professionals work in teams to address the complex and challenging needs of patients. Since this call, the Interprofessional Education Collaborative (IPEC) has been established [15]. One of the IPEC goals is to expand the Triple Aim. To date, this collaborative effort has been embraced by 21 professional healthcare organizations. Practically speaking, multiple healthcare professionals cannot be present for collaborative in-person visits with patients. Telehealth is the tool that eliminates the barrier of distance and time.

There will come a day when people will no longer be asking the question "can I use telehealth?" Instead, the question will be "when must I see the patient/doctor in person?" A time will come when telehealth technology will be fully integrated into every day clinical practice setting and every consumer devices. We will also see integration of telehealth technologies with electronic health records, which will be integrated with patient-generated health data, predictive analytics, and more. The full potential and power of this future vision, however, will not be realized until we are able to understand that the innovation is truly better than the idea that supersedes it; is consistent with the values and needs of clinicians and patients alike; is easy to understand and use; and has a venue for experimentation and whose use is visible on a regular basis. Much of this will need to start with our health professions training programs.

With the growing popularity of telehealth, telehealth training programs may become the new frontier in healthcare. A greater adoption of telehealth will spur healthcare training programs to incorporate didactic and experiential content into the curriculum. The National Organization of Nurse Practitioners has recently published a White Paper on the necessary components of telehealth education. The organization recommends that all nurse practitioners are trained in telehealth [16]. To date, only several schools of nursing have integrated telehealth into their curriculums. Beyond professional schools, most providers are receiving their telehealth training from vendors. Few training centers have been developed to prepare providers and healthcare organizations in telehealth. Without proper training, providers and centers often abandon telehealth leaving the perception that the industry is not ready for this type of healthcare delivery. As we move forward into the world of telehealth, policy and regulations should be maintained to assure safe and secure visits; yet we should assure that the regulations placed on this delivery is not overzealous and burdensome so that providers and patients alike will continue to adopt telehealth.

References

1. https://melnickmedicalmuseum.com/2009/12/01/a-short-history-of-stethoscopes.
2. Rogers EM. Diffusion of innovations. 5th ed. New York: Free Press; 2003.
3. Deloitte. 2018. https://www2.deloitte.com/insights/us/en/industry/health-care/virtual-health-care-health-consumer-and-physician-surveys.html.
4. Reinitis H, Teuss G, Bonney AD. Teaching telehealth consulting skills. Clin Teach. 2016;13(2):119–24.
5. Miller EA. The technical and interpersonal aspects of telehealth: effects on doctor patient communication. J Telemed Telecare. 2003;9(1):1–7.
6. Konath SH, O'Brien EH, Hsing C. Changes in dispositional empathy in American college students over time: a meta-analysis. Pers Soc Psychol Rev. 2011;15(2):180–98.
7. Bulik RJ. Human factors in primary care telehealth encounters. J Telemed Telecare. 2008;14:169–72.
8. American Telehealth Association. A concise guide for telehealth practitioners: human factors quick guide to eye contact. February 2016.

9. Edelson C. Virtual bedside manner: connecting with telehealth. Pediatric EHR Solutions. 2017. Retrieved from: https://blog.pcc.com/virtual-beside-manner-connecting-with-telehealth.
10. Major J. Using telemediquette to make your telehealth encounters effective. Arizona Telehealth Program. 2016. Retrieved from: telehealth.arizona.edu/blog/using-telemediquette-make-your-telehealth-enounters-effective.
11. Rheuban KS. Steps forward: support patient and care team coordination and communication through remote patient monitoring. Adopting telehealth in practice. American Medical Association. 2017. Retrieved from: https://www.stepsforward.org/modules/adopting-telehealth.
12. https://mhealthintelligence.com/news/telehealth-success-linked-to-workflow-rather-than-technology.
13. Lyles C, Sarkar U. Seeing the effect of health care delivery innovation in the safety net. JAMA Intern Med. 2017;177(5):649–50. https://doi.org/10.1001/jamainternmed.2017.0220.
14. https://www.healthitoutcomes.com/doc/the-road-to-mainstream-consumer-adoption-of-tele-health-0001.
15. Interprofessional Education Collaborative. Core competencies for interprofessional collaborative practice: 2016 update. 2016. Retrieved from: https://www.uab.edu/cipes/images/IP_Core_Competencies/IPEC-2016-Updated-Core-Competencies-Report__final_release_.PDF.
16. National Organization of Nurse Practitioners. NONPF supports telehealth in nurse practitioner education. 2018. Retrieved from: https://cdn.ymaws.com/www.nonpf.org/resource/resmgr/2018_Slate/Telehealth_Paper_2018.pdf.

Chapter 7
Telemedicine Quality and Quality Improvement in Pulmonary, Critical Care, Allergy, and Sleep Medicine

Elizabeth A. Brown and Jillian B. Harvey

Background on Quality in Health Care

Nearly twenty years ago, the Institute of Medicine released two landmark reports: "To Err is Human" and "Crossing the Quality Chasm" [1, 2]. These reports highlighted substantial problems associated with the quality of care in the United States. In *To Err is Human*, it was estimated between 44,000 and 98,000 hospital patients die each year from preventable medical errors [1]. The authors also estimated the United States annually spends between $17 and $29 billion in treatment costs related to preventable medical errors [1]. These reports emphasized the need for the US health care delivery system to make fundamental changes to address preventable medical errors and unnecessary costs [2]. Priority recommendations included the need for private and public purchasers, health care organizations, clinicians, and patients to work together to redesign health care processes [2].

The National Academy of Sciences states that the health care system does not function as well as it should and recommends both safety and effectiveness be improved [2]. While progress has been made within specific topic areas or within individual organizations, as a whole the US health care system continues to have major deficiencies related to access, cost, and quality.

E. A. Brown
Department of Health Professions, Medical University of South Carolina,
Charleston, SC, USA

J. B. Harvey (✉)
Department of Healthcare Leadership and Management, Medical University of South
Carolina, Charleston, SC, USA
e-mail: harveyji@musc.edu

© Springer Nature Switzerland AG 2021   109
D. W. Ford, S. R. Valenta (eds.), *Telemedicine*, Respiratory Medicine,
https://doi.org/10.1007/978-3-030-64050-7_7

Access

In a survey of patients, nearly 90% of the uninsured and 50% of privately insured report they have experienced a delay in care or were unable to get care due to financial reasons [3]. Examples of delays in care could include postponing appointments, treatments, and tests or reducing medication dosages without provider approval. Access challenges are especially problematic among patients living in rural or remote areas of the country, as many specialists and subspecialty providers reside in metropolitan areas [4]. For example, care management and triage for critically ill patients in community emergency departments can be extremely difficult for health care providers who may infrequently treat severe or specialized cases. This is heightened in pediatric critical care or trauma situations, where many community settings do not maintain critical care pediatric specialty providers or equipment for this population [5].

Cost

US health care spending continues to grow. In 2016, health care spending in the United States was $3.3 trillion, which accounts for nearly 18% of the gross domestic product (GDP) [6]. The GDP provides a proxy measure of a country's economic growth. Compared to other developed countries, the United States devotes a much higher percentage of the GDP to health care. Total US health care expenditures roughly equals spending $10,350 per person in the country [6]. Of this the majority of spending falls in three categories with hospital care services consuming the largest portion (32%), followed by physician and clinical services (20%), and prescription drugs (10%) [6].

Quality

In certain areas, gains have been made to the quality of care provided in the United States. For example, it is estimated the number of hospital-acquired conditions has declined by 1.3 million due to efforts of the Federal Partnership for Patients Initiative [7]. This public-private partnership brought together providers, employers, patients and government agencies to collaborate on initiatives designed to (1) make care safer and (2) improve care transitions [7]. However, severe problems persist, and there are many documented examples of how poor quality of care continues in both the inpatient and outpatient settings. Approximately 10% of patients experience an adverse event, defined as harms caused by the medical care diagnosis or treatment. Examples of adverse events include infection, falls, or adverse drug reactions [7]. Although patient safety and quality has been a major focus within hospitals for nearly two decades, studies now estimate that over 400,000 patients die each year in US hospitals due to preventable medical errors [8]. If deaths from medical errors were included on death certificates, "medical error" would be the third leading cause of death in the United States [9].

Structure, Process, and Outcomes in Health Care Quality

Before work can take place to improve patient care, the definition of quality and how it will be assessed must be addressed [10]. Several entities have defined health care quality and prioritized the areas of health care that need the most improvement. The US Agency for Healthcare Research and Quality defines health care quality as "doing the right thing, at the right time, in the right way, for the right person—and having the best possible results" [11, p. 735].

Donabedian Model The foundational framework to define and measure the components of health care quality were developed by Dr. Arvedis Donabedian. Donabedian recommended using the Structure, Process, Outcomes framework to assess the quality of care. Structure includes the elements that are essential to providing care (e.g., staff/provider qualifications, capital resources, human resources, organizational systems, technology, and policies). Process elements include the activities and interventions conducted to provide care. Finally, a variety of health care outcomes can be evaluated under this framework, including patient satisfaction, mortality, quality of life, and recovery. The three-part framework of structure, process, and outcome is important to understand because there are linkages between the three components. The underlying personnel or financial resources of the health care setting (structure) impact how the medical care is offered to patients (processes), which in turn affects patient outcomes such as in-hospital mortality or hospital-acquired infections. Thus, patient outcomes are directly related to structure and processes [10].

Quality Improvement Tools and Theory

Since the time of *To Err is Human,* it has become increasingly clear that the underlying issues related to patient safety and quality are complex systematic factors. To fully see widespread improvements, systematic and data-driven approaches to quality must be prioritized. Quality improvement includes any "systematic, data-guided activities designed to bring about immediate improvement in health care delivery in particular settings" [12].

The Model for Improvement

There are several commonly used methods to improve health care quality; these same methods can be used to improve care delivered through telehealth services. Continuous quality improvement (QI) seeks to improve processes, systems, and activities using data-driven approaches [13]. Quality assurance programs seek to manage areas defined by regulatory and accreditation organizations [14]. Health care providers have also adapted methods from other industries including Six Sigma, which attempts to reduce or eliminate errors and variation in processes while

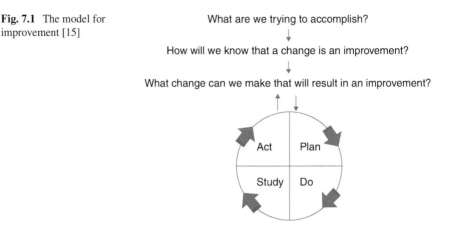

Fig. 7.1 The model for improvement [15]

elevating patient satisfaction and financial stability; and the Lean Production System, which focuses on identifying customer needs and removing processes that do not add value [14]. Another common approach is the Plan-Do-Study-Act (PDSA) cycle. This method plans small tests of change and then collects data to determine if the changes were successful. The process is analyzed and can be repeated through several cycles [15] (Fig. 7.1). Three primary questions guide improvement efforts in the PDSA cycle:

1. "What are we trying to accomplish?" Under this question, the team should identify goals for improvement, also known as aim statements. Aim statements should be written in a "SMART" format where the goal is *S*pecific, *M*easurable, *A*ctionable, *R*ealistic, and *T*imely [16]. The aim statement guides efforts and data collection and keeps the improvement work concise.
2. "How will we know a change is an improvement?" This question is where data sources and metrics are identified and examined. Data sources could include administrative data, interviews, surveys, observations, and electronic medical records. Consideration should be given to the availability and accuracy of the data sources [17]. In addition, this question seeks to identify what has historically happened that led to the situation. Tools in this stage should include data collection, analysis, and mapping or diagraming each step in the process to identify inefficiencies and potential causes of errors. The collected data should be utilized for a "root cause analysis" where the information is systematically assessed to identify factors that contribute to poor quality. One common root cause analysis tool is the "fishbone diagram," where the problem statement is listed at the far right of the diagram (Fig. 7.2). Next data-driven and brainstormed causes of the problem are categorized onto branches of the diagram. The branch category names can be customized to fit the specific problem. Each potential cause of the problem is explored asking "why does this occur?" This tool allows health care stakeholders to move beyond high-level assumptions and focus on actionable items. Figure 7.2 highlights how primary and secondary causes can be organized within a fishbone diagram to facilitate discussion among providers and further examination of the factors contributing to the problem [18].

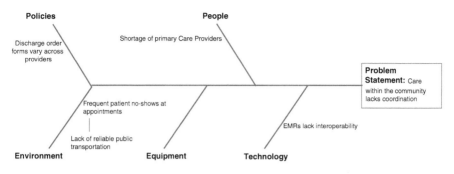

Fig. 7.2 Sample fishbone diagram

3. "What changes can we make that will result in improvement?" It is recommended to include front-line staff and those who can directly impact barriers and resources when making process improvement decisions. An interdisciplinary team should work together to recommend, explore, examine, and observe changes. After identifying possible changes, the team can prioritize possible improvement approaches.

These three questions combined with the PDSA cycle form what is known as "The Foundation for Improvement" [15] (Fig. 7.1). The PDSA cycle is used to develop, test, and implement changes. Repeated cycles are used to study the impact of small changes to processes, study the results, and respond accordingly. Specifically, in each step:

- Plan: Determine the changes to be implemented and design the improvement plan.
- Do: Implement the changes and document problems.
- Study: Examine the data and results. In this step, lessons can be learned from both successes and failures.
- Act: Make changes to the process based on lessons learned.

After completion of one cycle, the team should run additional PDSA cycles and implement successful changes into the standard care processes. Initial cycles can test feasibility of changes and test processes under differing circumstances.

Telehealth and Health Care Quality

As medical technology continues to advance, telehealth is one promising approach to improving cost, access, and quality of health care. Evidence supports that telehealth impacts on care through several mechanisms:

- Improved interactions across providers to improve care
- Facilitating provider-to-provider training
- Enhancing service quality and capacity

- Allowing direct provider to patient interaction, when the two are separated by time or space
- Managing patients with comorbid conditions from a distance
- Monitoring patient health and activities (e.g., home monitoring of blood pressures) [19]

Multi-Level Approaches to Quality Improvement and the Role of Telehealth

Given the multiple approaches to improving quality and the unlimited settings and scenarios telehealth services can be applied to, it is key to understand the role telehealth can play in facilitating QI. The community-level QI model has been described as a "family of concentric circles" with the patient residing in the center, and as one moves outward, the additional circles include those stakeholder groups who also have a responsibility toward the success or failure of the patient's care [10, 20, 21]. Given that telehealth work generally crosses traditional mechanisms of health care delivery, it is important to understand the QI interventions and approaches at each level.

Historically, QI efforts have targeted providers and organizations, ignoring the patient and caregiver's voice and the outer circle of community-level planning. It is believed that in order to make significant and sustainable changes in the health care system, activities must target all levels either simultaneously or incrementally. Simultaneous work does not mean that the same interventions must take place at each level, but that the goals and visions of each level must be coordinated and understood by all, and one level's work should not be counterproductive to the work of others [20, 21]. Improving the quality of care will require examination across all levels. Telehealth technology provides a tool to reach across the levels of the health care system to disseminate best practice and engage multiple stakeholders in patient care processes. When designing QI approaches, it is important to think about the multiple levels of the health care system and how telehealth can facilitate improvement efforts that can reach outside the boundaries of the traditional health care organization. It is possible this expanded approach to health care can overcome some of the challenges that have previously prevented population-level improvement in health outcomes [21].

Patient Level

Patient-level approaches include those focusing on the individual, such as patient education, health literacy, and other interventions created to engage the patient in their health and health care [21, 22]. Mobile technology such as apps, wearables, and patient home monitoring provide opportunities to engage the patient in the care processes. In addition, the data collected allows for improved patient-provider communication and decision-making.

Provider Level

At the provider level, QI methods typically focus on provider education, data feedback, and guideline adherence. Attempting to change the behaviors of individual providers previously had little effect on outcomes since providers may practice in several hospitals—each setting having its own requirements, policies, and procedures [10, 20, 21]. Therefore, telehealth technology can be leveraged to standardize care processes across care settings, and connect providers for consultation, education, and mentoring.

Group/Team Level

Many health care services are provided through a team. These teams consist of a variety of individuals including any combination of primary care physicians, specialists, nurses, allied health providers, social workers, or mental health providers and can work within one organization or across multiple settings. There is evidence that well-run teams provide higher quality care, but developing effective teams is a challenging task [20, 21]. Improving the quality and coordination of care provided by health care teams is becoming increasingly important due to the aging population and growing prevalence of chronic diseases, which require coordinated care across settings [20, 21]. Telehealth can facilitate team-based care through connecting teams who are otherwise distanced by physical space or time.

Organization Level

Health care quality assurance programs, collaboratives, regulatory/accreditation inspections, and continuous quality improvement are administered at the organizational level [14, 21]. Many of these collaboratives and interventions focus on organizational change and making care processes more efficient. However, these programs, sometimes, lack physician involvement and executive support. As a result, many telehealth programs are not sustainable or never move beyond the pilot stage [23]. Utilizing telehealth technology will require organizational support and a clear vision. Otherwise, there is a danger that the organization will move from project to project without disseminating learnings or achieving sustainable results. The most important factor in organizational-level quality is providing the culture for change and adapting to new insights [20, 21].

Community Level

To reduce missed opportunities, duplication of efforts, and unintended effects of the QI initiatives on the other levels of the health care system, patients, providers, groups, and organizations must have a way to communicate and understand what is taking place at each level. Through developing and implementing a community-level infrastructure, the telehealth technology can help disseminate information and coordinate QI work across settings. A community-wide approach could facilitate the diffusion of best practices and utilization of effective QI tools. Furthermore, certain factors (reimbursement, access, etc.) to improving quality are out of the control of individual providers or organizations and require a regional approach to impact quality [10, 21].

It is suggested that community QI efforts require careful planning and a strong infrastructure including the following characteristics: (1) a compelling vision and purpose, (2) a thoughtfully developed intervention, (3) strong management of the work, and (4) adequate resources [21, 24]. Telehealth systems that impact patient outcomes will require collaboration and evaluation across all the levels of the health care system.

Potential Impact of Telehealth on the Six Domains of Health Care Quality

In 2001, several goals to improve the quality of health care were outlined in the landmark report *Crossing the Quality Chasm*. These six domains of health care quality are a framework designed to minimize the number of preventable deaths and injuries in the medical community. All health care stakeholders, including policy-makers, purchasers, health care systems, consumers, and medical organizations and associations [2] should work together to address the six aims for improving health care quality. Here, in this section, we provide a broad overview of the IOM's six domains in relation to quality telehealth.

The six aims for improving health care [2]:

- Safe: Avoiding harm to patients from the care that is intended to help them
- Timely: Reducing waits and sometime harmful delays for both those who receive and those who give care
- Effective: Providing services based on scientific knowledge to all who could benefit and refrain from providing services to those not likely to benefit

- Efficient: Avoiding waste, including waste of equipment, supplies, ideas, and energy
- Equitable: Providing care that does not vary in quality because of personal characteristics such as gender, geographic location, and socioeconomic status
- Patient-centered: Providing care that is respectful of and responsive to individual patient preferences, and needs, and values

Safe: Avoid Injuries to Patients

Telehealth has the potential to impact measures of patient safety, such as preventing complications or, minimizing hazardous outcomes. The greatest potential impact of telehealth on patient safety is related to improving mortality outcomes. This may be especially true in certain medical professions such as critical care, emergency medicine, and neurology. For medical professionals who work with individuals with life-threatening conditions, such as heart failure, chronic obstructive pulmonary disease (COPD), renal failure, or stroke, there is evidence that telehealth can positively impact mortality rates. For example, tele-ICU services allow providers remote access to monitoring patient vital signs, laboratory results, and the ability to assist the bedside clinicians in interventions [25]. A tele-ICU program that provided remote ICU monitoring (12:00–07:00) to supplement traditional on-site ICU care was associated with a reduced risk of patient mortality during the period of remote ICU care [26–28]. At a minimum, it appears that telehealth could be equally as safe as in-person care. Several studies see no difference in mortality rates when implementing telehealth into critical care services [29, 30].

Telehealth technologies can also be used to increase safety and compliance of patient self-management. Several approaches to keeping patients safe during a telehealth visit include providing clear instructions, using safe equipment, and showing patients how to use equipment and medical devices. For example, pulmonary rehabilitation reduces disease severity and improves quality of life for patients living with COPD. However, due to workforce shortages and access issues, few patients complete the pulmonary rehab programs. Home-based tele-education and monitoring of stable COPD patients provide an opportunity for patients to undergo safe and supervised exercise training [31]. Participants use a specially designed cycle ergometer to increase safety during pulmonary rehabilitation exercises. Additionally, program assistants showed patients how use technological devices and how to properly sit on the cycle during exercises [31]. The impact of telehealth on patient safety may even go beyond traditional measures within the health care system. For example, patients of a tele-sleep program indicated that being provided sleep services at the local clinic allows access to care within the patient's community and reduces the chances of a motor vehicle accident as chances of auto accidents are typically higher in patients with sleep apnea [32].

Monitoring and educating providers within the clinical setting and patients within the home setting through telehealth systems can provide additional oversight and potentially mitigate the chance of errors. The potential increase in patient safety has been perceived by the health care workforce. For example, the percentage of ICU nurses who stated they would feel safe being treated in their ICU increased by 37% after implementation of a tele-ICU program. Nurses in another remote ICU monitoring program reported a greater than 50% increase in confidence that physician orders were correctly implemented and the perceived ability to reach an ICU physician greatly improved under tele-ICU [27]. In addition, as telehealth services are added to the health care system, this provides an opportunity to re-engineer services and standardize care processes. Telehealth systems can also facilitate patient safety through promoting communication across care teams and empowering individuals to intervene on patient safety concerns [27].

However, many telehealth programs do not outright address patient safety [33]. Telehealth programs should focus on ways to improve patient safety as well as eliminate provider or technological errors that may negatively impact patient outcomes. For instance, providers should examine if patients can safely participate in the telehealth program or intervention. This is especially important in direct to home/consumer telehealth programs, where the patient could be at risk of injuries such as falling. Additionally, telehealth programs should specifically track safety metrics (e.g., medication errors) and implement process improvement methods to avoid telehealth-related health care provider errors that could harm patients.

Timely: Reduce Waits and Harmful Delays for Those Who Receive and Provide Care

Care delivered through telehealth technology can reduce the amount of time it takes for patients to access health care services [34]. The improved access and time to treatment is one of the clearest benefits of telehealth services. The faster time to care can happen through several mechanisms. First, telehealth services may bring the care closer to the patient by using technology to service patients where they live and work. Telehealth services can reduce time spent waiting for specialty appointments, eliminate travel costs, and reduce travel times for patients [35]. Next, telehealth can facilitate rapid decision-making and consultation among providers through video-based conferencing, tele-monitoring, and store-and-forward technology. Under telehealth services, the consulting provider can have real-time access to view patients in a tele-ICU or receive alerts and intervene when congestive heart failure patients gain weight, or COPD patients have poor medication adherence. These early interventions may help to avoid emergency situations and unnecessary hospitalizations [34].

By reducing wait times, patients have better access to care. For example, children living with asthma, generally live in rural or underserved areas where specialty care is unavailable or limited; thus, telehealth care in asthma treatment may improve timely access to quality care [36]. Tele-presenters located with the asthma patient can perform spirometry, teach proper inhaler use, and manipulate the digital stethoscope and otoscope for remote examination of ears and nose. Likely due to improved time to treatment and elimination of travel burdens, compliance with asthma visits is often higher with telehealth services [36].

Timely access to care is not only beneficial for the patient but should also enhance the health care providers' experiences. In some cases, telehealth programs can reduce provider burden. For example, health care providers cited a decrease in clinical workload associated with a tele-sleep program [32]. Under a tele-ICU program, bedside nursing vacancy rates declined in over 80% of participating hospitals [27]. Many health care organizations experience turnover and provider shortages. Telehealth programs have shown increased provider satisfaction and reduced turnover rates, thus reinforcing patient access to timely care [27].

Effective: Provide Services Based on Scientific Knowledge to Avoid Underuse and Overuse

There is scientific literature on the effectiveness of telehealth care on various patient outcomes [36–38]. One caution is that many telehealth services have been developed and implemented within the care delivery system without the scrutiny of randomized clinical trials. Providers should utilize the highest level of scientific evidence and practice guidelines when providing care through telehealth technologies.

The implementation of quality telehealth programs may have a positive impact on patient health outcomes. In a 2012 Cochrane Review and meta-analysis of 10 randomized controlled trials, researchers found telehealth did not improve quality of life for COPD patients; however, researchers noted a decrease in the odds ratio of emergency department admissions and hospitalization [38]. In critical care studies, scientists have found that intensive care telehealth can reduce mortality, length of stay, and costs to care for the critically injured [27]. Specifically, remote ICU consultations have shown to reduce ICU mortality and length of stay [39]. In another study where researchers compared asthma outcomes in children, participants appeared to have better control of asthma with telehealth [36]. Remote monitoring of asthma patients is associated with a reduction in hospitalizations over a 12-month period [35, 40].

In many cases, remote telehealth services are not intended to replace but to meaningfully supplement bedside care. The added layer of supervision provided through telehealth allows specialty providers to visualize the patient rather than relying on verbal information over the telephone. Store-and-forward technologies and remote home monitoring provide additional access to patient data. Through these mechanisms, telehealth can provide opportunities for early intervention and improved patient outcomes.

Efficient: Avoid Waste (Equipment, Supplies, Ideas, and Energy)

Demand for many health care services is increasing. Severe shortages of specially trained providers, uneven geographic dispersion of providers [27], increased elderly population, and increasing patient morbidity all contribute to patient demand for care. If the health care system is unable to sufficiently increase the supply of providers, then in order to meet treatment demands, the system must become more efficient. As previously mentioned, telehealth provides opportunities to reduce time to care, travel costs, and productivity loss from missed work or school, thereby making the provision of care more efficient for the patient. For providers, telehealth combined with Electronic Health Record (EHR) systems may facilitate the collection of health information, which could reduce time and energy spent researching information elsewhere. For example, providers may be alerted to abnormal patient vital signs or poor medication adherence. Quick access to credible information may deter adverse medical events and complications. Furthermore, the telehealth technology can minimize provider time spent physically traveling between clinics or units. To maximize the potential efficiencies, telehealth providers should utilize quality improvement and lean techniques to minimize the amount of waste within care processes [34].

The primary concern related to telehealth is that the evidence base is primarily focused on the potential efficiencies to the system and the impact of telehealth services on access and process measures. Therefore, there is a lack of cost-effectiveness data for telehealth services [35]. The lack of appropriate measures and quality data appears to be concern across several disciplines when examining cost-effectiveness in telehealth. More data are needed to determine the cost-effectiveness of telehealth care in asthma care [40]. In 2015, for those with sleep apnea, researchers found that telehealth was cost-effective, resulting in lower costs and a minimal loss of productivity [37]. In another study, telehealth in the ICU appeared to be cost-effective; however, authors noted the lack of transparent cost data and the minimal number of studies examining cost-effectiveness [30]. Additionally, researchers noted a reduction in ICU costs [28], cost per case [26], and costs of care [27] when using telehealth in the critical care setting. Yet, in a 2010 study, researchers found no reduction in hospital costs when examining the impact of a telehealth program in an ICU unit [29]. Undoubtedly, there is a need for more cost-effective studies that provide better insight to the effect of telehealth on cost outcomes.

Equitable: Provide Quality Care That Does Not Vary Based on Characteristics Like Gender, Race/Ethnicity, Location, and/or Socioeconomic Status

One of the primary benefits of telehealth is the ability to provide equitable services to diverse populations with varying health conditions irrespective of patient location. The goal of telehealth must be to provide care that does not vary in quality based on patient or provider characteristics [34].

Through telehealth services, patients in rural and remote settings have increased opportunities to receive certain types of care than may otherwise be accessible. For example, telehealth sites allow patients to be seen by specialty providers without having to travel great distances [35]. Telehealth technology can also be used to overcome language barriers through tele-interpreter services. Innovative technology utilization can also be used to connect providers with traditionally difficult to reach patient populations. For example, young adults with asthma are less likely to have a routine source of care and may rely on emergency services. Therefore, compliance with treatment is low and often results in increased morbidity and mortality [41]. Targeted use of telehealth and mobile technologies within certain populations can reduce disparities in access and outcomes and promote equitable health care delivery.

Patient-Centered: Providing Respectful and Responsive Care to Each Individual Based on Patient Values

The driving force behind providing care via telehealth should be patient-centered. Telehealth is designed to improve access to care and reduce barriers to treatment by providing care where patients reside. The benefits of telehealth are reduced barriers to care for patients, care coordination, and enhanced patient-provider communication. Reports of patient satisfaction across multiple telehealth services remain high [32, 36]. To promote patient-centered care, telehealth providers should consider patient preferences, values, and needs during the care process [34].

Telehealth Measurement and Outcomes

Due to the unique data challenges of telehealth delivery in the real-world setting, telehealth research and evaluation requires innovative data collection and analysis techniques [42]. Telehealth programs often begin as pilot programs or small-scale supplements to in-person care. In recent situations of natural disaster or pandemics, telehealth services may be rapidly implemented to maintain health care delivery during times of reduced travel and social distancing. Traditional measurement guidance may assume a fully implemented service and do not take into consideration these small-scale and staged developments in telehealth implementation. As a result, many telehealth programs rely on simple counts of programmatic data, while others pursue advanced analysis (e.g., cost-effectiveness), without having appropriate sample sizes.

The applied telehealth measurement framework adapts the National Quality Forum's (NQF) telehealth measurement domains, program evaluation, and telehealth maturity models to create a measurement tool for telehealth service evaluation and improvement [19, 43, 44]. The National Quality Forum has identified four domains of telehealth outcomes that program administrators/providers should be collecting and analyzing. These domains include the following: (1) access to timely care and appropriate health care based on the patient's needs; (2) financial impact and cost of telehealth; (3) patient and clinician experience; and (4) effectiveness of the system, clinical care, and technology. Within each measurement domain, telehealth processes and outcomes may mirror the metrics collected in traditional care. The metrics selected under each domain should be evidence based, valid, and reliable [10]. The model recommends outcome domains for each stage of program maturity and provides guidance on data sources, program evaluation, and research methods. The model is intended to be generalizable to all types of telehealth service modalities (synchronous, asynchronous, store-and-forward, remote patient monitoring, etc.), as well as adaptable to telehealth service lines or disease condition. Starting with Stage 0, the program leaders should plan for future data collection needs and evaluation. As the telehealth service grows, more advanced measures and evaluation techniques can be deployed. Stage 3 aims to assess the population-level impact of the telehealth service. Table 7.1 provides an example of how guideline-based care and the NQF framework for telehealth care can be assessed and is grounded in proposed levels of telehealth program maturity. Applying this type of framework can help enable telehealth programs to match their metrics and evaluation approaches with the scope/scale of their programs.

Conclusion and Future Directions

There is evidence that telehealth can improve access to care, quality outcomes, and cost-effectiveness. However, major disparities still exist within the US health care system, and providers and systems are not routinely adopting evidence-based practice in general. To overcome the challenges within the health care system, telehealth can be strategically integrated to enhance quality. The Agency for Healthcare Research and Quality (AHRQ) defines three aims to improve health care in the future, and it is important to consider the potential role of telehealth within each aim:

1. *Achieving better care.* Appropriately used telehealth is ideally situated to facilitate both improvement of patient process and dissemination of best practices across organizations. This will require collaboration and implementation of significant changes to culture and practice. In many cases, health care organizations fail to apply the scientific improvement tools discussed in this chapter. Furthermore, lessons learned and effective best practices are often not disseminated beyond the original source and rarely reach across organizations. The health care community needs to embrace quality and safety as a core value [7]. Clinicians must understand and utilize quality improvement strategies including the PDSA cycle.
2. *Achieving healthy people and communities.* Telehealth is a promising approach to improving care and alleviating the issues causing morbidity and mortality.

Table 7.1 Applied Telehealth Measurement Framework-Outcome

Stage	0: Pipeline – service feasibility	1: Pilot exploration	2: Established program	3: Optimization
Definition/ criteria	Stakeholder needs are identified and program feasibility is explored. Service model and technology are selected *Problem being targeted must be defined in a quantifiable way*	Service is tested on a small scale and iteratively refined based on real-world experience *Workflow is established Pilot is ready for growth*	Standard operating procedures are in place *Service is maintaining expected volumes and is sustainable*	Program is at scale and is sustainable *Population impact can be measured*
Measure domains	Feasibility Organizational readiness Resource availability Demand Cost/payment Benefit	Utilization Process measures Service specific measures Satisfaction Technical quality Leadership and stakeholder buy-in Cost (NQF)	Effectiveness Availability of care Risk-adjusted utilization Patient and clinician experience (NQF)	Access to care (NQF) Value-based outcomes Cost-effectiveness (NQF) Population-level outcomes
Potential data sources	Qualitative data Publicly available health outcomes and cost Surveys Organizational operational and financial data *These data also used in later stages	Qualitative data Electronic health records Patient registries Program-specific tracking logs Billing records	Claims data Electronic health records Patient registries Program-specific tracking logs Prospective data collection protocols	Claims data Electronic health records Patient registries Program-specific tracking logs Prospective data collection protocols
Quality management tools and study design	Quality and strategic planning Needs assessment Literature reviews Process/workflow mapping	Quality improvement (PDSA, run charts, fishbone, root cause) Program evaluation and descriptive studies *Pilot clinical trials when appropriate	Quality improvement, cross-sectional analysis, pre-/post-analysis, cohort and case-control studies, quasi-experimental, multi-center trials, natural experiment, pragmatic trials *Clinical trials when appropriate	Quality control (dashboarding, benchmarking, control charts); cohort and case control studies; quasi-experimental; multi-center trials; natural experiment; pragmatic trials *Clinical trials when appropriate

However, to impact population-level health outcomes, a community-level approach to quality improvement and sharing of best practices must be embraced. This includes reducing barriers to care and eliminating disparities based on geography, race, ethnicity, gender, socioeconomic status, age, sex, and other determinants of health. More attention needs to be paid to any potential negative consequences of telehealth or potential harms [39].

3. *Making care affordable.* A considerable benefit of telehealth is reduced patient travel time and expenses. However, little evidence exists regarding the financial impact of telehealth on the health care system. When implementing and evaluating telehealth services, particular attention should be paid to measures of process efficiency and reducing waste. Furthermore, providers should be cautious of increased utilization of telehealth services that provide little benefit to the patient.

References

1. Institute of Medicine. To err is human. Washington, DC: National Academies Press; 2000.
2. Institute of Medicine. Crossing the quality chasm: a new health system for the 21st century. Washington, DC: National Academies Press; 2001.
3. Agency for Healthcare Research and Quality. National healthcare quality and disparities report. Rockville: Agency for Healthcare Research and Quality; 2017. AHRQ Pub. No. 17-0001.
4. American Academy of Pediatrics: Task force on regionalization of pediatric critical care. Consensus report for regionalization of services for critically ill or injured children. Pediatrics. 2000;105:152–5.
5. Athey J, Dean M, Ball J, et al. Ability of hospitals to care for pediatric emergency patients. Pediatr Emerg Care. 2001;17(3):170–4.
6. Centers for Medicare and Medicaid Services. National Expenditure 2016 Highlights. 2016. https://www.cms.gov/Research-Statistics-Data-and-Systems/Statistics-Trends-and-Reports/NationalHealthExpendData/Downloads/highlights.pdf Accessed 25 June 2020.
7. National Patient Safety Foundation. Free from harm: accelerating patient afety improvement fifteen years after to err is human. Boston: National Patient Safety Foundation; 2015.
8. James JTA. A new, evidence-based estimate of patient harms associated with hospital care. J Patient Saf. 2013;9:122–8. https://doi.org/10.1097/PTS.0b013e3182948a69. pmid:23860193.
9. Makary M. Medical error-the third leading cause of death in the US. BMJ. 2016;353:i2139.
10. Donabedian A. The quality of care: how can it be assessed? J Am Med Assoc. 1988;260(12):1743–8.
11. Varkey P, Reller MK, Resar RK. Basics of quality improvement in health care. Mayo Clin Proc. 2007;82(6):735–9.
12. Lynn J, Baily MA, Bottrell M, Jennings B, Levine RJ, Davidoff F, et al. The ethics of using quality improvement methods in health care. Ann Intern Med. 2007;146:666–73.
13. Robert Wood Johnson Foundation. The science of continuous quality improvement. 2014. https://www.rwjf.org/en/library/research/2012/06/improving-the-science-of-continuous-quality-improvement-program-0.html Accessed 25 June 2020.
14. Hughes RG. Tools and strategies for quality improvement and patient safety. Patient safety and quality: an evidence-based handbook for nurses. 3rd ed. Rockville: Agency for Healthcare Quality and Research; 2008.
15. Langley G, Nolan K, Nolan T. The foundation of improvement. Quality Progress. ASQC. 1994: 81–86.

16. Ogrinc GS, Joint Commission Resources Inc, Institute for Healthcare Improvement. Fundamentals of health care improvement: a guide to improving your patient's care. 2nd ed. Cambridge, MA: Institute for Healthcare Improvement; 2012.
17. Murphy D, Ogbu O, Coopersmith C. ICU Director Data: using data to assess value, inform local change, and relate to the external world. Chest. 2015;147(4):1168–78.
18. American Society for Quality. Learn about quality: Fishbone diagram. 2020. https://asq.org/quality-resources/fishbone. Accessed 25 June 2020.
19. National Quality Forum (NQF). Creating a framework to support measure development for telehealth. Funded by the Department of Health & Human Services Contract HHSM-500-2012-000091, Task Order HSM-500-T0022. 2018.
20. Ferlie EB, Shortell SM. Improving the quality of health care in the United Kingdom and the United States: a framework for change. Milbank Q. 2001;79(2):281–315.
21. Harvey J. Evaluating community level approaches to improving healthcare outcomes. (Doctoral Dissertation). Available from ProQuest database. 2014.
22. Leatherman S, Sutherland K. Designing national quality reforms: a framework for action. Int J Qual Health Care. 2007;19(6):334–40.
23. AlDossary S, Martin-Khan MG, Bradford NK, Armfield NR, Smith AC. The development of a telemedicine planning framework based on needs assessment. J Med Syst. 2017;41(5):7–4. https://doi.org/10.1007/s10916-017-0709-4.
24. Perla RJ, Bradbury E, Gunther-Murphy C. Large-scale improvement initiatives in healthcare: a scan of the literature. J Healthcare Quality. 2013;35(1):30–40. Retrieved from http://onlinelibrary.wiley.com/doi/10.1111/j.1945-1474.2011.00164.x/abstract
25. Kahn JM, Hill NS, Lilly CM, Angus DC, Jacobi J, Rubenfeld GD, et al. The research agenda in ICU telemedicine: a statement from the Critical Care Societies Collaborative. Chest. 2011;140(1):230–8. https://doi.org/10.1378/chest.11-0610.
26. Breslow MJ, Rosenfeld BA, Doerfler M, Burke G, Yates G, Stone DJ, et al. Effect of a multiple-site intensive care unit telemedicine program on clinical and economic outcomes: an alternative paradigm for intensivist staffing. Crit Care Med. 2004;32(1):31–8. https://doi.org/10.1097/01.CCM.0000104204.61296.41.
27. Groves RH, Holcomb BW, Smith ML. Intensive care telemedicine: evaluating a model for proactive remote monitoring and intervention in the critical care setting. Stud Health Technol Inform. 2008;131:131–46.
28. Rosenfeld BA, Dorman T, Breslow MJ, Pronovost P, Jenckes M, Zhang N, et al. Intensive care unit telemedicine: alternate paradigm for providing continuous intensivist care. Crit Care Med. 2000;28(12):3925–31.
29. Morrison JL, Cai Q, Davis N, Yan Y, Berbaum ML, Ries M, Solomon G. Clinical and economic outcomes of the electronic intensive care unit: results from two community hospitals. Crit Care Med. 2010;38(1):2–8. https://doi.org/10.1097/CCM.0b013e3181b78fa8.
30. Venkataraman R, Ramakrishnan N. Outcomes related to telemedicine in the intensive care unit: what we know and would like to know. Crit Care Clin. 2015;31(2):225–37. https://doi.org/10.1016/j.ccc.2014.12.003.
31. Holland AE, Hill CJ, Rochford P, Fiore J, Berlowitz DJ, McDonald CF. Telerehabilitation for people with chronic obstructive pulmonary disease: feasibility of a simple, real time model of supervised exercise training. J Telemed Telecare. 2013;19(4):222–6. https://doi.org/10.1177/1357633X13487100.
32. Hirshkowitz M, Sharafkhaneh A. A telemedicine program for diagnosis and management of sleep-disordered breathing: the fast-track for sleep apnea tele-sleep program. Semin Respir Crit Care Med. 2014;35(5):560–70. https://doi.org/10.1055/s-0034-1390069.
33. Schlachta-Fairchild L, Elfrink V, Deickman A. Patient safety, telenursing, and telehealth. In: Hughes RG, editor. Patient safety and quality: an evidence-based handbook for nurses. Rockville: Agency for Healthcare Research and Quality; 2008.
34. Schwamm L. Telehealth: seven strategies to successfully implement disruptive technology and transform health care. Health Aff. 2014;33(2):200–6.

35. Goodridge D, Marciniuk D. Rural and remote care: overcoming the challenges of distance. Chron Respir Dis. 2016;12(2):192–203.
36. Portnoy JM, Waller M, De Lurgio S, Dinakar C. Telemedicine is as effective as in-person visits for patients with asthma. Ann Allergy Asthma Immunol. 2016;117(3):241–5. https://doi.org/10.1016/j.anai.2016.07.012.
37. Isetta V, Negrín MA, Monasterio C, Masa JF, Feu N, Álvarez A, Campos-Rodriguez F, Ruiz C, Abad J, Vázquez-Polo FJ, Farré R. A Bayesian cost-effectiveness analysis of a telemedicine-based strategy for the management of sleep apnoea: a multicentre randomised controlled trial. Thorax. 2015;70(11):1054–61. https://doi.org/10.1136/thoraxjnl-2015-207032.
38. McLean S, Nurmatov U, Liu JL, Pagliari C, Car J, Sheikh A. Telehealthcare for chronic obstructive pulmonary disease: Cochrane review and meta-analysis. Br J Gen Pract. 2012;62(604):e739–49. https://doi.org/10.3399/bjgp12X658269.
39. Totten AM, Hansen RN, Wagner J, Stillman L, Ivlev I, Davis-O'Reilly C, Towle C, Erickson JM, Erten-LyonsD, Fu R, Fann J, Babigumira JB, Palm-Cruz KJ, Avery M, McDonagh MS. Telehealth for acute and chronic care consultations. Comparative effectiveness review no. 216. (Prepared by Pacific Northwest Evidence-based Practice Center under Contract No. 290-2015-00009-I.) AHRQ Publication No. 19-EHC012-EF. Rockville, MD: Agency for Healthcare Research and Quality; April 2019. Posted final reports are located on the Effective Health Care Program search page. https://doi.org/10.23970/AHRQEPCCER216.
40. McLean S, Chandler D, Nurmatov U, Liu J, Pagliari C, Car J, Sheikh A. Telehealthcare for asthma: a cochrane review. CMAJ. 2011;183(11):E733–42. https://doi.org/10.1503/cmaj.101146.
41. MacDonell K, Naar S, Gibson-Scipio W, Bruzzese J, Wang B, Brody A. The Detroit young adult asthma project: Proposal for a multicomponent technology intervention for African American emerging adults with asthma. JMIR. 2019;7(5):e98.
42. Tuckson RV, Edmunds M, Hodgkins ML. Telehealth. N Engl J Med. 2017;377(16):1585–92.
43. National Committee for Quality Assurance. HEDIS Measures across 6 domains of care. 2020. https://www.ncqa.org/hedis/. Accessed 25 June 2020.
44. Van Dyk L, Schutte SL. The telemedicine service maturity model: a framework for the measurement and improvement of telemedicine services. Rijeka: IntechOpen; 2013. https://doi.org/10.5772/56116.

Part II
Telehealth in Pulmonary, Critical Care, Allergy and Sleep Medicine

Chapter 8
Telehealth for Pediatric Asthma

Claire A. MacGeorge, Annie Lintzenich Andrews, and Kathryn L. King

Introduction

Clinical Vignette

DF is an otherwise healthy 8-year-old male with past medical history of asthma requiring hospitalization, most often during the winter months. His grandmother often keeps him home from school due to his symptoms, leading to poor academic performance. His primary care physician prescribed albuterol and fluticasone, but he has not been able to make it to a visit for 9 months. He regularly visits his school nurse for rescue albuterol, but this year he does not have the proper paperwork on file at school to allow the nurse to legally administer this medication. So, when DF presented to the nurse's office today wheezing and the nurse was unable to reach his grandmother, her only available course of action was to call 911 and have him transported to the local emergency room.

Asthma is one of the most common and costly chronic diseases of childhood affecting 10% of children. It is associated with significant morbidity and high rates of school absenteeism. In fact, asthma is one of the top reasons children ages 5–17 are absent from school, with approximately 36,000 children missing school because of their asthma each day [1]. One study estimated that medical costs, loss of work, and missed school days account for a total economic burden of more than $81.9 billion annually [2].

Fortunately, effective medications are available to prevent and treat the symptoms of this chronic condition. Appropriate use of controller medications, primarily

C. A. MacGeorge · A. L. Andrews · K. L. King (✉)
Department of Pediatrics, Medical University of South Carolina, Charleston, SC, USA
e-mail: kingkl@musc.edu

© Springer Nature Switzerland AG 2021
D. W. Ford, S. R. Valenta (eds.), *Telemedicine*, Respiratory Medicine,
https://doi.org/10.1007/978-3-030-64050-7_8

inhaled corticosteroids, can reduce asthma exacerbations, acute care visits for asthma, and hospitalizations [3, 4]. However, significant barriers exist to children receiving effective therapy. In particular, children from minority as well as low-income families in both inner-city and rural areas encounter significant barriers to asthma care resulting in greater rates of poorly controlled asthma and preventable emergent health care utilization [5–7].

Telehealth has been shown to be a valuable tool in overcoming these barriers to pediatric asthma care. Telehealth modalities, including live video visits, asynchronous visits, and remote patient monitoring, have been used to provide patient and provider education, monitor symptoms, and assess medication adherence and inhaler technique. These telehealth programs have led to improvement in asthma-related health outcomes, increased access to care, and cost-effectiveness [8].

In this chapter, we describe the application of various telehealth modalities to pediatric asthma and explore the role of school-based telehealth in managing pediatric asthma.

Application of Telehealth Modalities to Pediatric Asthma

Telehealth provides a unique opportunity to provide care for children with asthma in a more patient-centered manner. Telehealth modalities used in pediatric asthma care include real-time live video (synchronous), store-and-forward (asynchronous), remote patient monitoring, and mobile health (mHealth). Real-time live video involves clinician to patient contact using video at the same time while store-and-forward involves a clinician reviewing information provided by a patient at a different point in time. Remote patient monitoring is a specific type of store-and-forward that collects data over time for cumulative review. Mobile health can be either synchronous or asynchronous but involves the use of mobile phone technology in health care. Figure 8.1 provides an overview of telehealth modalities, types of asthma care services, and associated outcomes.

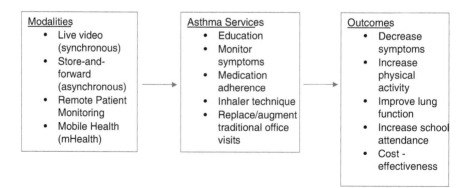

Fig. 8.1 Telehealth modalities for delivering asthma services and associated outcomes

Real-Time Live Video (Synchronous) Pediatric Asthma Care

Real-time live video visits are a secure, real-time, two-way interaction between a patient and a clinician using remote audiovisual technology. For asthma care, this modality has been used to diagnose asthma, to prescribe treatment, and to provide patient education with mixed results. A study in *Journal of Asthma* showed that a brief video intervention offered during pediatric clinic visits led to immediate improvements in children's inhaler techniques, though the change was not sustained [9]. A comprehensive asthma education program delivered by telehealth in rural Arkansas was able to improve monitoring of symptoms and medication adherence but did not change quality of life, self-efficacy, asthma knowledge, or lung function [10].

Additionally, the Extension for Community Healthcare Outcomes (ECHO) Model was delivered by the University of New Mexico in 2003 as a platform to deliver specialty care education to primary care providers in rural areas. Using a virtual hub-and-spoke model, community clinicians in rural areas are connected to experts at academic health centers through co-management of patients and didactic sessions. Specifically, for asthma care, education was provided for respiratory therapists, nurses, and clinicians at community hospitals [11]. Since its inception, it has been implemented across the nation. While specific outcome studies on the use of this platform for pediatric asthma have not been performed, a systematic review including 39 studies concluded Project ECHO is an effective and potentially cost-saving model that increases participant knowledge and patient access to health care in remote locations [12].

Store-and-Forward (Asynchronous) for Pediatric Asthma Care

Store-and-forward telehealth includes the transmission of patient data, recorded videos, and digital images such as X-rays and photographs via secure communication systems to a health care provider, who can then review this information and provide recommendations and advice at a later time. A randomized trial of children with persistent asthma examined the combined effects of asynchronous review of history and physical exam with physician/caregiver follow-up and school nurse-administered controller medication. This study design highlights the multiple added efficiencies of school-based telehealth and found that the intervention group had significantly more symptom-free days and fewer emergency department visits [13].

Remote Patient Monitoring for Pediatric Asthma Care

Remote patient monitoring involves medical data collection from an individual in one location via electronic communication technologies, which is transmitted to a provider in a different location for use in patient care and support. In a multi-center, randomized controlled trial with a 16-month follow-up conducted in the Netherlands, children with asthma had 50% of their visits replaced with virtual visits. They received online care using a virtual asthma clinic with 8 monthly outpatient visits with monthly web-based monitoring in addition to usual care. The visits were performed at the school with a telemedicine assistant either with live videoconference or by gathering symptom data to be stored and transmitting to their primary care practice if telemedicine. Clinicians reviewed the visit within 3 days and contacted the caregiver via phone or videoconference. Compared to controls, the children receiving the monitoring had significantly more symptom-free days (difference of 1.23 days, $p = 0.0003$) and improved asthma control as measured on the asthma control test, prompting the authors to conclude that routine outpatient visits can partially be replaced by monitoring children with asthma through telehealth [14].

Mobile Health for Pediatric Asthma Care

Mobile health (mHealth) has been shown to be an innovative way to incorporate self-management into care plans. Using mHealth application (apps), patients are able to receive educational information and reminders, track symptoms, and communicate symptom information to health care providers. Although most studies have been conducted among adolescents and adults with asthma, they have generally shown positive effects in clinical (e.g., asthma control), patient-reported (e.g., medication adherence and quality of life), and economic outcomes (health care visits) [15]. A recent study using a mobile application called Smartphone Asthma Monitoring System tracked inhaler use as measured by a blue-tooth cap showed that families found this to be an acceptable means of reporting symptoms and medication use. Data were transmitted on 89% of study days [16]. Screenshots of the patient view associated with this asthma management app are provided in Fig. 8.2 and illustrate the approach to tracking medication adherence and asthma education options.

Medical Societies Support Telehealth for Asthma Management

As telehealth programs have expanded across the nation, key organizations have endorsed position statements in support of telehealth for the management of pediatric asthma. This includes the American Academy of Pediatrics (AAP) and the American College of Allergy, Asthma, and Immunology (ACAAI).

The AAP specifically endorses the use of telemedicine to address access and physician workforce shortages. In the 2015 position statement, they highlight how the AAP can advocate for physicians and patients to optimize telemedicine to

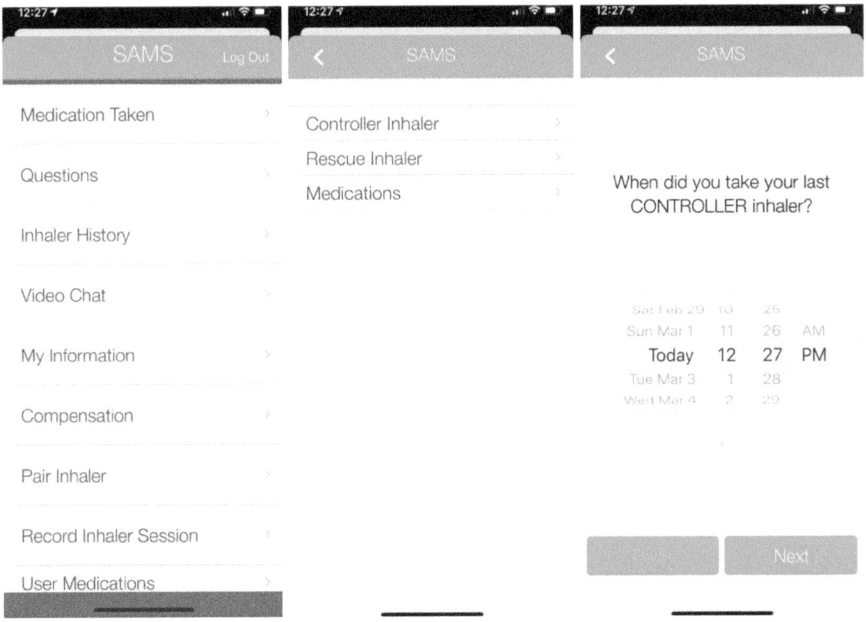

Fig. 8.2 Smartphone Asthma Monitoring System is an example of an mHealth technology that enables a clinician to receive real-time information regarding a patient's asthma symptoms

improve access to care, provide more patient- and family-centered care, increase efficiencies in practice, enhance the quality of care, and address projected shortages in the clinical workforce [17].

The American College of Allergy, Asthma, and Immunology advocates for the incorporation of meaningful and sustained use of telemedicine in allergy and immunology practice [8]. Additionally, they support the use of telehealth, particularly citing the importance of having a professional with a specialization in asthma involved in patient care. The organization recognizes that a large proportion of the asthma burden lies among patients in underserved communities and that telehealth can help relieve barriers to care created by distance and provider shortages [8].

Asthma Care in School-Based Telehealth

After home, school is the location where children spend the majority of their time. An estimated 50 million children in the United States spend a significant portion of their day in school, making this venue an ideal place for health interventions [18]. School-based health centers are clinics staffed by qualified health care professionals that provide quality, comprehensive health services in a school during school hours. There are currently over 2500 school-based health clinics that provide primary care onsite or using telehealth by a qualified health professional. In the case of asthma care specifically, school-based interventions have been shown to be effective in reducing asthma symptoms, and improving activity, lung function, asthma understanding/knowledge, missed school days, ED visits, and hospitalization to varying degrees [19].

There is inherent benefit to schools from investing in asthma-related interventions. The evidence for the link between asthma and academic achievement is so robust that it was chosen as the second of seven strategic priorities by an expert review panel for the *Journal of School Health*'s Special Issue on "Healthier Students are Better Learners" in 2011 [18]. Within this special issue, authors highlighted that childhood asthma effects multiple educational outcomes including, "cognition, connectedness with engagement in school, and absenteeism, and the effects of comorbidity such as sleep disruption and multiple risk factors on ability to succeed in school" [20]. However, it was also noted that while school-based interventions have the potential to reduce both educational and health disparities, these efforts are not well supported at the public health level.

Within the schools providing asthma care, there has been a marked increase in those providing care through telehealth, a practice, which is well-supported in the literature. The percentage of school-based health centers using telehealth has more than doubled from 7% in 2007–2008 to 19% in 2016–2017 [21]. Romano et al. observed a cohort of 17 patients treated in a rural school-based clinic who received follow-up care via telehealth after an initial in-person visit. The authors found that reported symptom scores, quality of life, and FEV_1 improved similarly to those of patients who received face-to-face care [22]. Additionally, a study of 40 patients receiving care for asthma via telehealth over a series of 3 visits found no difference in care between the telehealth and control group and interestingly found a higher dropout rate among the control group who had to travel for appointments [23]. These small feasibility studies have helped garner financial support for larger programs and paved the way for more robust work. A recent study published in *JAMA Pediatrics* showed that a school-based, asthma-focused telehealth program in a rural county in South Carolina was associated with a 21% relative decrease in the likelihood of ED visits among a subsample of children with asthma [24]. Throughout the 6-year study period, the effect size increased annually indicating that the degree of success may evolve over time because of the additive effect of learning experience of participants. This emphasizes the need for uptake to occur to increase both the utilization and impact of school-based telehealth. This finding is supported by an additional study showing that children participating in a school-based telemedicine enhanced asthma management program in Rochester, New York, had more symptom-free days and were less likely to have an emergency department visit or hospitalization for asthma compared with controls (odds ratio = 0.52) [13].

The key to success of school-based telehealth often involves engaging a wide variety of stakeholders necessary for a comprehensive asthma care. More specifically, these interventions have typically included community health providers in educational programs for students, staff, and families or increasing the amount of clinical care available at school through supporting and extending the hours of school nurses, establishing school-based health centers, and offering mobile clinics [25–27]. The reviews emphasize the importance of engaging families, community resources, primary care physicians, and school nurses as key stakeholders that each plays a vital role in the ecological framework of this complex health care issue. Special emphasis must be placed on connecting these stakeholders in order to help families navigate the unique circumstances that are involved in managing asthma at school such as having a documented asthma management plan available in addition to both rescue and controller medication. One study found that rates of asthmatic students having a quick-relief inhaler at school range from 14% to 39% with rates of accompanying physician's orders, parental permission, and a documented management plan even lower [28].

As school-based telehealth has become a reality for more and more children across the country, it has also garnered support from professional organizations and the evidence base for its benefits has increased. The American Telemedicine Association's Operating Procedures for Pediatric Telehealth, which were published and endorsed by the AAP in 2017, support the use of school-based telehealth services and in particular highlight the use of telehealth for chronic pediatric diseases such as asthma. These operating procedures outline minimum guidelines for safety and quality of care in this setting and our delineated in Table 8.1 [29].

Clinical Vignette Follow-Up

Upon returning to school in the fall, the school nurse had identified DF as a "high risk asthmatic" following asthma training/education she had just received over the summer. DF's grandmother completed and returned the consent forms to enroll him in the school-based health program. He was seen by a provider early in the school year, prior to experiencing an asthma exacerbation, his asthma severity was assessed and the best asthma management plan for him was determined. When DF presented to the nurse acutely wheezing, she is able to request a visit with a nurse practitioner who gathers a history via video and performs a lung exam via a peripheral stethoscope. An order for albuterol from the clinician's telehealth stock is given to the school nurse. DF receives the albuterol treatment, is reassessed by the provider via telehealth, and is returned to class, allowing him to resume learning in a timely fashion. Asthma education is provided to the patient and family, prescriptions are sent to the pharmacy, and a note is sent to DF's primary care physician.

Table 8.1 Best practices for school-based telehealth

Agreements and consents	Agreements executed between school district and provider Consents include HIPAA[a], FERPA[b], and consent to treat Consents are signed prior to a visit taking place
Technology	Complete IT[c] assessment at both the school site and provider site prior to selecting equipment Utilize a HIPAA compliant platform and adhere to HITECH[d] regulations Test equipment prior to going live Provide ongoing IT support
Training	School nurse or telepresenter must be trained in equipment operation and how to conduct the exam Provider must be privileged and appropriately trained to conduct visits via telehealth Scope of services should be outlined
Visits	Obtain appropriate medical history and medical home information Allow parents to participate in the visit either in person, by phone or video Contact parent following the visit if he/she does not participate Ensure HIPAA and FERPA compliance throughout visit Avoid distractions during the visit Ensure that patient and provider have been introduced and that all persons present during the visit are acknowledged Ensure that the standard of care is maintained
Medical home	Ensure timely and thorough communication with the medical home following every visit

[a]Health Insurance Portability and Accountability Act of 1996
[b]Family Educational Rights and Privacy Act
[c]Information Technology
[d]Health Information Technology for Economic and Clinical Health Act

Key Components of Quality Asthma Care in Schools

Best Practices for School-Based Health

In order to provide high quality care to children in schools using telehealth, a structured protocol should be in place to ensure each child receives comprehensive, guideline-driven care while maintaining patient privacy and supporting the medical home. Best practices for each of the components of care are highlighted in Table 8.1 and described in detail below.

Process of Care

Either written or digital consent is obtained from a parent, usually at the start of the school year. When the patient presents to the school nurse for evaluation, a parent is contacted. The visit with an "on-call provider" is requested and within 15 minutes, the patient is connected to a provider via video. Any necessary treatments can be done in the nurse's office with an order from the provider. Any needed prescriptions

Fig. 8.3 School-based telehealth workflow. (1) Consent forms are signed. (2) Patient presents to school nurse for evaluation, visit is determined to be necessary, and parent is contacted. (3) Telehealth visit takes place. (4) Patient returns to class. (5) Prescriptions (as needed) are sent to local pharmacy. (6) Communication is sent to PCP

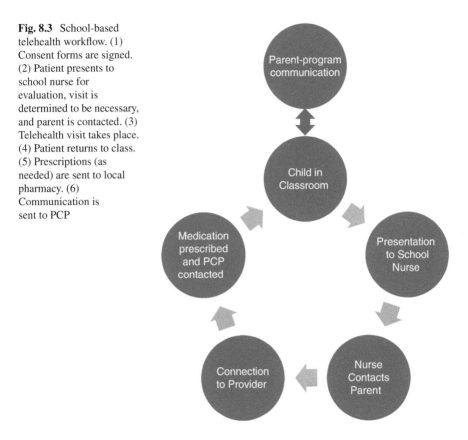

can be sent to either a pharmacy designated by the family or one that delivers to the school. Communication is sent to the primary care physician (See Fig. 8.3 and Table 8.1.)

Equipment

A provider connects to the school nurse through a Health Insurance Portability and Accountability Act – compliant video conferencing platform and assesses the child. History is obtained from the school nurse and the patient, and telemedicine peripheral devices including a digital stethoscope, otoscope, and exam camera are used to conduct a thorough assessment of the child's condition in real time.

The Role of School Nurses in Asthma Care

The importance of the function of the school nurse is repeatedly emphasized in the literature as they often play a key role in communication between school staff, medical providers, and families and are on the frontline of school-based public health strategies. Formally engaging school nurses in asthma case management has been shown to be associated with students being more likely to have medication at school, use a peak flow meter, and have an improvement in pulmonary function [28, 30]. However, school nurses are often not fully supported or utilized in school-based asthma care with lack of time, education, and communication cited as common barriers [31]. These barriers can be particular challenges for school nurses located in rural areas, where provider shortages can make their involvement even more necessary. In a survey of school nurses in both urban and rural areas, Carpenter et al. found that while most had some asthma training, school nurses in rural schools were much less likely to have received this support and almost all would have liked to have additional training [31].

Engagement of Parents, Teachers, and Primary Care Physicians

A crucial component of comprehensive asthma care is involvement of all the key stakeholders in a child's care. While school-based telehealth overcomes barriers related to working parents by allowing some care to be delivered in their absence, communication with parents, including the delivery of asthma education, is essential to symptom control outside of school. Likewise, teachers are often the frontline of detecting symptoms in children, prompting referral to the school-based health clinic and should be taught identification of children needing referral for diagnosis or management of asthma. Finally, as school-based health clinics are designed to augment and not replace primary care providers, written or verbal summaries of visits should be communicated to the medical home.

Potential Barriers to Asthma Management by Telehealth

While many studies have shown the benefit of asthma management using telehealth, particularly in the school-based health setting, barriers exist to its effective implementation in the clinical setting. Because comprehensive asthma care necessitates the engagement of many stakeholders, programs must be well-designed and deployed. In addition to school nurses and school-based personnel, parents and school administrators must be engaged and supportive of the time and resources needed for the endeavor. Because parents may not be in attendance for visits, obtaining consent and communicating changes in plan can be a challenge. Additionally, alternative plans for care while school is not in session for holidays and summer must be determined. Another common theme identified in school-based health literature is lack of sustainability of such programs. Often grant funded, any additional employees or support for school nurses tends to end with the funding period, and sustaining involvement from busy clinicians must ultimately involve a sustainable reimbursement structure [25, 27].

Financial Considerations

Importantly, payment models that reflect prevention and early intervention would greatly enhance the viability of school-based interventions. However, while value-based payment models are being deployed for the pediatric population, they are often focused on metrics that are designed for clinic-based care. The newest payment models for remote patient monitoring and virtual check-ins that are currently being piloted in adult populations also hold promise for the school-based application. Future program evaluations and payment advocacy should be focused on metrics that encourage contact points with patients more frequently than the clinic-based care model allows in order to build on current successes. For example, tracking of symptoms proactively could be done in the school setting, as could repeat education to make sure children have optimal compliance with medications.

Conclusion

Despite a number of logistical barriers and a need to expand the evidence base, the future is bright for school-based telehealth interventions for asthma. It will become increasingly important to leverage a population-based approach in order to reach the right children at the right time with the right intervention and maximize cost-effectiveness. Utilizing multiple telehealth modalities, such a remote patient monitoring for medication adherence and symptom tracking and asynchronous and video visits involving the school nurse and asthma professionals, has the potential to provide a truly team-based approach. The convenience of school-based care combined with the increased patient contact provided by telehealth has the potential to provide wrap around care that will best serve children with asthma and their families and help to decrease the physical, educational, and financial impact of this disease.

Telehealth provides a unique opportunity to overcome typical barriers in providing asthma care to children. Modalities such as real-time video visits, store-and-forward, remote patient monitoring, and mobile health have been used to provide patient and provider education, monitor symptoms and medication adherence as well as assess inhaler technique, and even replace typical office visits. In particular, school-based telehealth has been shown to be effective in reducing asthma symptoms, improving physical activity, lung function, asthma understanding/knowledge, missed school days, ED visits, and hospitalization.

References

1. Zahran HS, Bailey CM, Damon SA, Garbe PL, Breysse PN. Vital signs: asthma in children – United States, 2001–2016. MMWR Morb Mortal Wkly Rep. 2018;67(5):149–55.
2. Nurmagambetov T, Kuwahara R, Garbe P. The economic burden of asthma in the United States, 2008–2013. Ann Am Thorac Soc. 2018;15(3):348–56.

3. Adams RJ, Fuhlbrigge A, Finkelstein JA, et al. Impact of inhaled antiinflammatory therapy on hospitalization and emergency department visits for children with asthma. Pediatrics. 2001;107(4):706–11.

4. Sin DD, Man SF. Low-dose inhaled corticosteroid therapy and risk of emergency department visits for asthma. Arch Intern Med. 2002;162(14):1591–5.

5. Lin NY, Ramsey RR, Miller JL, et al. Telehealth delivery of adherence and medication management system improves outcomes in inner-city children with asthma. Pediatr Pulmonol. 2020;55(4):858–65.

6. Lintzenich A, Teufel RJ, Basco WT Jr. Under-utilization of controller medications and poor follow-up rates among hospitalized asthma patients. Hosp Pediatr. 2011;1(1):8–14.

7. Valet RS, Gebretsadik T, Carroll KN, et al. High asthma prevalence and increased morbidity among rural children in a Medicaid cohort. Ann Allergy Asthma Immunol. 2011;106(6):467–73.

8. Elliott T, Shih J, Dinakar C, Portnoy J, Fineman S. American college of allergy, asthma & immunology position paper on the use of telemedicine for allergists. Ann Allergy Asthma Immunol. 2017;119(6):512–7.

9. Carpenter DM, Lee C, Blalock SJ, et al. Using videos to teach children inhaler technique: a pilot randomized controlled trial. J Asthma. 2015;52(1):81–7.

10. Perry TT, Halterman JS, Brown RH, et al. Results of an asthma education program delivered via telemedicine in rural schools. Ann Allergy Asthma Immunol. 2018;120(4):401–8.

11. Arora S, Kalishman S, Dion D, et al. Partnering urban academic medical centers and rural primary care clinicians to provide complex chronic disease care. Health Aff (Millwood). 2011;30(6):1176–84.

12. Zhou C, Crawford A, Serhal E, Kurdyak P, Sockalingam S. The impact of project ECHO on participant and patient outcomes: a systematic review. Acad Med. 2016;91(10):1439–61.

13. Halterman JS, Fagnano M, Tajon RS, et al. Effect of the school-based telemedicine enhanced asthma management (SB-TEAM) program on asthma morbidity: a randomized clinical trial. JAMA Pediatr. 2018;172(3):e174938.

14. van den Wijngaart LS, Roukema J, Boehmer ALM, et al. A virtual asthma clinic for children: fewer routine outpatient visits, same asthma control. Eur Respir J. 2017;50(4):1700471.

15. Farzandipour M, Nabovati E, Sharif R, Arani MH, Anvari S. Patient self-management of asthma using mobile health applications: a systematic review of the functionalities and effects. Appl Clin Inform. 2017;8(4):1068–81.

16. Teufel Ii RJ, Patel SK, Shuler AB, et al. Smartphones for real-time assessment of adherence behavior and symptom exacerbation for high-risk youth with asthma: pilot study. JMIR Pediatr Parent. 2018;1(2):e8.

17. Committee On Pediatric W, Marcin JP, Rimsza ME, Moskowitz WB. The use of telemedicine to address access and physician workforce shortages. Pediatrics. 2015;136(1):202–9.

18. Basch CE. Healthier students are better learners: a missing link in school reforms to close the achievement gap. J Sch Health. 2011;81(10):593–8.

19. Al Aloola NA, Naik-Panvelkar P, Nissen L, Saini B. Asthma interventions in primary schools--a review. J Asthma. 2014;51(8):779–98.

20. Basch CE. Asthma and the achievement gap among urban minority youth. J Sch Health. 2011;81(10):606–13.

21. Adams NL, Rose TC, Elliot AJ, et al. Social patterning of telephone health-advice for diarrhoea and vomiting: analysis of 24 million telehealth calls in England. J Infect. 2019;78(2):95–100.

22. Romano MJ, Hernandez J, Gaylor A, Howard S, Knox R. Improvement in asthma symptoms and quality of life in pediatric patients through specialty care delivered via telemedicine. Telemed J E Health. 2001;7(4):281–6.

23. Portnoy JM, Waller M, De Lurgio S, Dinakar C. Telemedicine is as effective as in-person visits for patients with asthma. Ann Allergy Asthma Immunol. 2016;117(3):241–5.

24. Bian J, Cristaldi KK, Summer AP, et al. Association of a school-based, asthma-focused telehealth program with emergency department visits among children enrolled in South Carolina Medicaid. JAMA Pediatr. 2019;173(11):1041–8.

25. Cicutto L, Gleason M, Szefler SJ. Establishing school-centered asthma programs. J Allergy Clin Immunol. 2014;134(6):1223–30.
26. Taras H, Wright S, Brennan J, Campana J, Lofgren R. Impact of school nurse case management on students with asthma. J Sch Health. 2004;74(6):213–9.
27. Hollenbach JP, Cloutier MM. Implementing school asthma programs: lessons learned and recommendations. J Allergy Clin Immunol. 2014;134(6):1245–9.
28. Hanley Nadeau E, Toronto CE. Barriers to asthma management for school nurses: an integrative review. J Sch Nurs. 2016;32(2):86–98.
29. McSwain SD, Bernard J, Burke BL Jr, et al. American telemedicine association operating procedures for pediatric telehealth. Telemed J E Health. 2017;23(9):699–706.
30. Suwannakeeree P, Deerojanawong J, Prapphal N. School-based educational interventions can significantly improve health outcomes in children with asthma. J Med Assoc Thail. 2016;99(2):166–74.
31. Carpenter DM, Estrada RD, Roberts CA, et al. Urban-rural differences in school nurses' asthma training needs and access to asthma resources. J Pediatr Nurs. 2017;36:157–62.

Chapter 9
Ambulatory Telemedicine: Home-Based COPD Management

Gustavo Adolfo Fernandez Romero and Gerard J. Criner

Background

Chronic obstructive pulmonary disease (COPD) is a leading cause of death worldwide and is estimated to affect more than 16 million people in the United States [1]. Exacerbations of COPD cause a significant burden on the healthcare system in terms of costs, quality of life (QOL), disease progression, and mortality [2].

Telehealth, defined as a remote delivery of healthcare services and clinical information using telecommunications technology, involves a variety of devices (smartwatch, telephone, tablet, computers) and systems directed to increase access, provide convenience, and reduce cost. It is a rising component of healthcare with the potential to transform the way medicine has been practiced; nevertheless, the disparity in reimbursement is one of the major limitations [3, 4]. A European Respiratory Society task force proposed a series of definitions to describe the different telemedicine systems and unify criteria for the use of this technology that is summarized in Table 9.1 [5].

In the management of chronic diseases such as diabetes and hypertension, the use of telehealth has been demonstrated in randomized controlled trials (RCTs) and meta-analyses to be superior when compared to usual care for the control of outcomes such as hemoglobin A1C and blood pressure, respectively [6–8].

COPD is a complex disease due to the heterogeneity of clinical presentation, co-existing comorbidities, management and prognosis. The use of telemedicine has promise, but multiple studies and RCT's report conflicting outcomes associated with a variety interventions. As a result, there is presently insufficient evidence to recommend telehealth compared to usual care for the prevention of exacerbations,

G. A. Fernandez Romero (✉) · G. J. Criner
Department of Thoracic Medicine and Surgery, Lewis Katz School of Medicine at Temple University, Temple University Hospital, Philadelphia, PA, USA
e-mail: gustavo.fernandezromero@tuhs.temple.edu

© Springer Nature Switzerland AG 2021   143
D. W. Ford, S. R. Valenta (eds.), *Telemedicine*, Respiratory Medicine,
https://doi.org/10.1007/978-3-030-64050-7_9

Table 9.1 Definitions and applications

Telemedicine	Distribution of health services in conditions where distance is a critical factor by healthcare providers that use information and communication technologies (ICT) to exchange information useful for diagnosis at distance
Telecommunications	Use of cable connections, radio, optical means, or other electromagnetic channels to transmit or receive signals, such as voice, data, or video communications
Teleconsultation	Second opinion on demand between patient/family and staff or among health operators; opinions, advice provided at distance between two or more parties separated geographically
Telemonitoring	Digital/broadband/satellite/wireless or Bluetooth transmission of physiological and other noninvasive data (i.e., biological storage data transfer)
Decision support systems	According to a sentinel value, an alert starts for health personnel, who call patient
Remote diagnosis	Identifying a disease by the assessment of the data transmitted to the receiving party through instrumentation monitoring a patient away from the clinic
Tele-evaluation	On-demand data transfer to use as biological outcome measures
Telecare	Network of health and social services in a specific area; in case of emergency, patient calls medical personnel, emergency call service, or members of family
Telerehabilitation	Allows reception of homecare and guidance on the process of rehabilitation through connections for point-to-point video conferencing between a central control unit and a patient at home
Telecoaching	Direct reinforcement or recorded messages/communications to improve adherence
Teleconference, audio	Electronic two-way voice communication between two or more people located in different places

hospitalizations, mortality, or improvement of QOL among patients with COPD [9–11]. This chapter provides a review of the existing evidence for the use of telehealth in the home-based management of COPD.

Current State of Telehealth in COPD

Evidence for the use of telehealth in the management of COPD is variable and sometimes contradictory. A major reason is the variability in what the authors describe as the telehealth intervention under investigation. Some studies describe telehealth as monitoring of symptoms only, others as monitoring of biological variables (e.g., lung function, heart rate, respiratory rate, and pulse oximetry), and still others as enhanced communication between healthcare platforms. Very few studies have used telehealth applications to intervene in a structured format to improve patient care, or truncate the development of worsening exacerbation symptoms. Therefore, substantial differences between the various interventions, data collection, and applications do not permit rigorous comparisons between the studies to evaluate their impact on patient outcomes [11].

Bourbeau reported a multicenter, randomized, parallel-group, clinical trial done in 7 hospitals from Canada with a 1-year follow-up. The primary objective was to evaluate the impact of a self-management program and the ongoing telecommunication with a healthcare provider on the use of hospital services and QOL. They included the patients >50 years, with stable COPD (no changes in the medications in prior 4 weeks), current or previous smoker (at least 10 PPY), FEV_1/FVC <70, and FEV_1 between 25% and 70% and excluded patients with comorbidities such as CHF, dementia, terminal disease, history of asthma, and long-term hospitalizations. Patients were randomized into the intervention group or the control group. The intervention consisted of an education program on a disease-specific self-management program (1 h per week for 7–8 weeks) supervised by nurses, respiratory therapists, and physiotherapists who acted as case managers directed by the primary pulmonologists and followed by monthly telephone calls over a 12-month period. A total of 191 patients were randomized, 96 in the intervention group and 95 into the usual care. Hospital admissions were reduced by 39.8% in the intervention group ($p = 0.01$) versus the usual care, ED visits were reduced by 41% ($p = 0.02$), and unscheduled physician visits by 58.9% ($p = 0.03$), also improving the QOL scores at 4 months although some of the benefits were seen only for the 12 months duration of the study [12].

The Pennsylvania Study of COPD Exacerbations (PA-SCOPE) was a randomized, single-blinded, parallel-group trial with 24 months follow-up. It is one of the very few studies that has used a bidirectional asynchronous communication platform to provide a scripted tele-intervention based on an individual worsening of patient's respiratory symptoms and/or lung function using accepted guidelines of care. The primary end point was the number of hospitalizations and mortality. Eligible patients were between 40 and 80 years of age, current or former smokers with COPD diagnosis, and at least one hospitalization in the prior year or home oxygen use. The patients with significant comorbidities were excluded. After baseline evaluations, the patients were randomized to either the intervention group or the control group. All patients were instructed to document their symptoms with an electronic daily diary application (app) on a handheld device. The app had eight screens of questions that took 2–3 min to complete. They also obtained daily peak flow readings with a disposable peak flow meter. The patients in the control group that had worsening of disease were supposed to call their primary physician and follow their standard of care plan and the intervention group were instructed to call a 1-800 number if the symptoms algorithm reached or exceeded the predetermined threshold. The communication for the intervention group was available 24/7, and staffed by nurses and pulmonologists; the exacerbations were managed according to GOLD Report recommendations. A total of 79 patients were randomized; 39 to the intervention group and 40 to the control group. The demographic and clinical data showed that the groups were well matched. The intervention group patients had a higher compliance rate in daily diary reporting compared with control group patients (81.4% vs. 69.9%, respectively; $p < 0.001$); no serious adverse events were reported in either group. There was no difference in the hospitalization rates (number of hospitalizations/study observation days) (intervention group vs. control group, 35/10,951 vs. 44/12,012, respectively; $p = 0.63$), time to first hospitalization, mortality, and QOL. There was improvement in the daily symptoms and activity reported by the patients in the intervention group especially dyspnea ($p < 0.0006$) and peak flow improvement ($p < 0.0001$) that was sustained throughout the 24 months of follow-up. A reduction in the number of hospitalizations and exacerbations was observed in both groups but lacked power to demonstrate a difference in hospitalization rate or mortality between groups. The authors concluded that early interventions using telehealth decreased the development of subsequent exacerbations, decreased dyspnea, and improved peak flow and daily activity status [13].

McLean and colleagues published a promising Cochrane review and meta-analysis about telehealth for COPD. It included ten randomized controlled trials (RCT) from 211 articles identified in the literature search from different countries (the United States, Canada, Italy, Spain, Hong Kong, and Belgium) that met the validation criteria with a total of 1004 patients. Some of the studies relied on video-conferencing or the telephone as a basis for telecommunication. The use of telemedicine did not improve QOL mean difference in St Georges Questionnaire at 12 months −6.57 (95% confidence interval [CI] = −13.62 to –0.48) or mortality (OR = 1.05; 95% CI = 0.63–1.75), but there was a significant reduction in the emergency department visits (OR = 0.27; 95% CI = 0.11–0.66) and hospitalization (OR = 0.46; 95% CI = 0.33–0.65) [14].

A systematic review by Gregersen et al. addressed the question whether telehealth interventions improve the quality of life of patients with COPD, and it included 18 studies (1636 patients) but only three trials were found to have statistical significance supporting the use of telemonitoring. The authors recognize the inability to determine a quantitative synthesis due to the heterogeneity of the low number of studies [15].

Vittaca and colleagues published a literature review that included several databases (EMBASE, CINALH, PubMed, PsychINFO, and Scopus) for studies published since 2003–2017 and found 395 papers from which 46 RCT were included for analysis. The author grouped the studies according to the results into three groups: positive (4366 patients), contradictory (1259 patients), or negative (5699 patients) results. The patients were comparable with similar mean FEV_1 and frequent COPD exacerbations. They concluded from this heterogeneous group of studies that the best telemonitoring outcomes are expected in older and sicker populations with frequent exacerbations, multiple comorbidities, and limited community support; in addition, the best results came from programs using what they defined as third-generation telemonitoring that includes decision-making support led by a physician and full therapeutic authority 24/7 [16].

The PROMETE II Trial (Madrid Project on the Management of Chronic Obstructive Pulmonary Disease with Home Telemonitoring) was a multicenter, unblinded, randomized controlled trial of 12 months duration. The primary aim was to decrease the number of exacerbations leading to ED visits and hospital admission. They included patients with ages between 50 and 90 years old, diagnosed with

COPD, severe airflow obstruction (FEV1 < 50%), on home oxygen that had 2 or more moderate or severe exacerbation in the prior year, but clinically stable at the moment of the study (defined as 6 weeks without clinical symptoms). After providing the necessary equipment, the patients were trained on how to monitor their blood pressure, oxygen saturation, heart rate, and spirometry; the respiratory rate and oxygen saturation would be automatically obtained from the device attached to the home oxygen. After collecting 4 days of baseline parameters, an alert configuration was set. The information was received and a triage application graded patient reports according to the severity. A total of 229 patients were randomized into the home telemonitoring (115 patients) versus the routine clinical practice (RCP) (114 patients). There were no statistically significant differences in the proportion of patients who had a severe exacerbation leading to a hospital admission or an ED visit over 12 month period (60% vs. 53.5% in RCP $p = 0.321$). There was also no difference in the mean total of exacerbations, time to first exacerbation, daily activity, quality of life, or mortality. This study highlights the limitations in using telehealth systems based only on physiological parameters to identify acute COPD exacerbations in a timely manner and thus prevent the need for hospitalization or healthcare services [17].

Another trial using telemonitoring of physiological variables to identify and reduce severe exacerbations was recently published by Parker and colleagues. The CHROMED (Telemonitoring in Chronic Obstructive Pulmonary Disease) trial was a multicenter, randomized clinical trial, with a 9-month follow-up. The main objective was to determine the efficacy of home monitoring lung mechanics by the forced oscillation technique (FOT) and cardiac parameters. It included patients older than 60 years, with a diagnosis of COPD GOLD grade II or higher, a history of acute exacerbation with or without hospitalization in the previous 12 months, and at least one or more comorbidities. A total of 312 patients were randomized, usual care (158 patients) and telemonitoring (TM) (154 patients). The patients in the treatment group measured their lung mechanics daily using a device that measured FOT, a touch-screen computer and a mobile modem. An algorithm would trigger an alarm system and a call to identify the early need of interventions. This study did not find any changes in the time to first hospitalization, antibiotic prescriptions, hospitalization rate, or quality of life. An exploratory subgroup analysis of patients with higher risk in the telemonitoring group had fewer hospital readmissions [18].

Future Directions and Limitations

Further research is needed to understand if and how telehealth can improve the outcomes in the management of COPD. There is a need to standardize the telehealth interventions and data collection with the use of telemonitoring to better predict and intervene on acute exacerbations.

In general, use of telemonitoring that only captures physiologic parameters is inadequate to identify COPD exacerbations in the early phases and thus often too

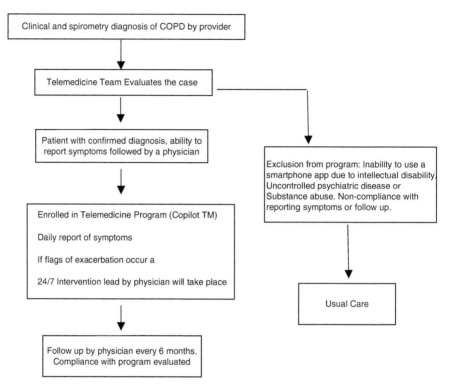

Fig. 9.1 COPD telemedicine protocol

late for meaningful intervention beyond emergency department and/or hospital use. Telehealth should be coupled with self-management approaches where patients that report worsening of their respiratory symptoms can be identified and timely, stepwise interventions offered that might better prevent the need of ED visits or hospitalizations. Below is offered a protocol in use at our organziation that comp-bines physiologic and patient-reported measures (Fig. 9.1).

COPD is a complex, heterogeneous disease where the majority of patients have multiple comorbidities. Telehealth interventions should also aim to control comor-bidities such as heart failure, diabetes, and anxiety/depression to prevent all-cause readmissions.

There are barriers to the use of telehealth in COPD such as experience with technological devices; education; and cognitive, motor, psychological, and visual abilities or deficits. Another aspect to be aware is cost of this technology, or reim-bursement for the clinical services provided. The recognition of patients that would benefit from this intervention should include the evaluation of these limita-tions [5].

References

1. NHLBI COPD National Action Plan. Available at: https://www.nhlbi.nih.gov/health-topics/education-and-awareness/COPD-national-action-plan. Accessed Oct 2018.
2. Shah T, Press VG, Huisingh-Scheetz M, White SR. COPD readmissions: addressing COPD in the era of value-based health care. Chest. 2016;150(4):916–26. https://doi.org/10.1016/j.chest.2016.05.002.
3. About telemedicine. Washington, DC: American Telemedicine Association. http://www.americantelemed.org/main/about/about-telemedicine/telemedicine-faqs.
4. Dorsey ER, Topol EJ. State of telehealth. N Engl J Med. 2016;375:154–61. https://doi.org/10.1056/NEJMra1601705; PMID: 27410924.
5. Ambrosino N, Vagheggini G, Mazzoleni S, et al. Telemedicine in chronic obstructive pulmonary disease. Breathe (Sheff). 2016;12:350–6.
6. Tchero H, Kangambega P, Briatte C, Brunet-Houardard S, Retali G-R, Rusch E. Clinical effectiveness of telemedicine in diabetes mellitus: a meta-analysis of 42 randomized controlled trials. Telemed J E Health. 2019;25(7):569–83.
7. Lee SWH, Chan CKY, Chua SS, Chaiyakunapruk N. Comparative effectiveness of telemedicine strategies on type 2 diabetes management: a systematic review and network meta-analysis. Sci Rep. 2017;7:12680. https://doi.org/10.1038/s41598-017-12987-z.
8. Margolis KL, Asche SE, Dehmer SP, et al. Long-term outcomes of the effects of home blood pressure telemonitoring and pharmacist management on blood pressure among adults with uncontrolled hypertension follow-up of a cluster randomized clinical trial. JAMA Netw Open. 2018;1(5):e181617.
9. Vogelmeier CF, Criner GJ, Martínez FJ, et al. Global strategy for the diagnosis, management, and prevention of chronic obstructive lung disease 2017 report: GOLD executive summary. Eur Respir J. 2017;49:1700214.
10. Criner GJ, Bourbeau J, Diekemper RL, et al. Prevention of acute exacerbations of COPD: American College of Chest Physicians and Canadian Thoracic Society Guideline. Chest. 2015;147:894–942.
11. Bourbeau J, Farias R. Making sense of telemedicine in the management of COPD. Eur Respir J. 2018;51:1800851. https://doi.org/10.1183/13993003.00851-2018.
12. Bourbeau J, Julien M, Maltais F, et al. Reduction of hospital utilization in patients with chronic obstructive pulmonary disease a disease-specific self-management intervention. Arch Intern Med. 2003;163(5):585–91. https://doi.org/10.1001/archinte.163.5.585.
13. Cordova FC, Ciccolella D, Grabianowski C, et al. A telemedicine-based intervention reduces the frequency and severity of COPD exacerbation symptoms: a randomized, controlled trial. Telemed J E Health. 2016;22(2):114–22. https://doi.org/10.1089/tmj.2015.0035.
14. McLean S, Nurmatov U, Liu JL, et al. Telehealthcare for chronic obstructive pulmonary disease: cochrane review and meta-analysis. Br J Gen Pract. 2012;62:e739–49.
15. Gregersen TL, Green A, Frausing E, et al. Do telemedical interventions improve quality of life in patients with COPD? A systematic review. Int J Chron Obstruct Pulmon Dis. 2016;11:809–22.
16. Vitacca M, Montini A, Comini L. How will telemedicine change clinical practice in chronic obstructive pulmonary disease? Ther Adv Respir Dis. 2018;12:1753465818754778.
17. Ancochea J, García-Río F, Vázquez-Espinosa E, et al. Efficacy and costs of telehealth for the management of COPD: the PROMETE II trial. Eur Respir J. 2018;51:1800354. https://doi.org/10.1183/13993003.00354-2018.
18. Walker PP, Pompilio PP, Zanaboni P, et al. Telemonitoring in COPD: the CHROMED study, a randomized clinical trial. Am J Respir Crit Care Med. 2018;198:620. https://doi.org/10.1164/rccm.201712-2404OC.

Chapter 10
Home-Based Evaluation and Management of Sleep Disordered Breathing via Telehealth

Chitra Lal and Akram Khan

Abbreviations

AASM	American Academy of Sleep Medicine
CBOC	Community-Based Outpatient Clinics
CPAP	Continuous positive airway pressure
CVT	Clinical Video Telehealth
HSAT	Home sleep apnea testing
OSA	Obstructive sleep apnea
PAP	Positive end-airway pressure
PSA	Patient services assistant
RP	Respiratory polygraphy
SDB	Sleep disordered breathing
TM	Telemedicine
VAMC	Veterans Affairs Medical Center

Introduction

Sleep disordered breathing (SDB) is increasingly being recognized as a common clinical problem in primary care [1]. The demand for specialized care for SBD and other sleep-related problems is increasing with a declining number of

C. Lal (✉)
Department of Pulmonary, Critical Care, Allergy and Sleep Medicine, Medical University of South Carolina, Charleston, SC, USA
e-mail: lalch@musc.edu

A. Khan
Department of Pulmonary Critical Care, Oregon Health & Sciences University, Portland, OR, USA

© Springer Nature Switzerland AG 2021
D. W. Ford, S. R. Valenta (eds.), *Telemedicine*, Respiratory Medicine,
https://doi.org/10.1007/978-3-030-64050-7_10

board-certified sleep physicians [2]. The population of the United States is approximately 325 million as estimated by the United States Census Bureau. According to the American Academy of Sleep Medicine (AASM), there are approximately 7500 board-certified sleep specialists indicating that the ratio of people to sleep specialists in the United States is more than 43,000:1 [2]. Data from AASM also show geographical barriers with board-certified sleep physicians and accredited sleep centers clustering in more urban, highly populated areas [2]. Sleep providers have been using asynchronous telemedicine (TM) with home sleep apnea testing (HSAT) and positive end-airway pressure (PAP) adherence monitoring in routine practice for many years [3]. The convenience of telemedicine is especially noteworthy for the management of chronic illnesses such as SDB as many patient visits can be conducted remotely utilizing a secure HIPPA compliant system without sacrificing quality of care [3–6].

As long as appropriate technical standards are met and roles and responsibilities of various providers are clearly defined, a TM-based approach has great potential in improving access to care, reducing wait times as well as costs [4, 5, 7]. Implementation of a comprehensive sleep TM protocol has been shown to increase the volume of sleep consultations, volume of sleep testing while reducing the time between consultation and PAP prescriptions, thus improving access to care [4, 5, 7]. An analysis of 5695 visits to a Veterans Affairs Medical Center (VAMC) between 2005 and 2013 showed that patients saved 142 minutes per visit and 145 miles of travel on average [8]. There was a modest reduction in costs to the healthcare system due to reduction in travel payments. The implications of such an approach for public health policy are significant, and enthusiasm about the use of TM in sleep medicine has reached a point that the American Academy of Sleep Medicine (AASM) has produced a position paper for the use of TM for the diagnosis and treatment of sleep disorders [3].

There are studies showing improved adherence to PAP at 3 months with a TM-based approach [9, 10] as well as decreased delay to the first technical intervention in PAP-treated patients. As short-term PAP adherence has been shown to predict adherence at 1 year, improving short-term adherence to PAP with a TM-based approach may also improve long-term adherence. Telemonitoring is also well received by the majority of patients although a few have found it to be intrusive [11, 12].

The shortage of sleep-trained workforce, increasing recognition of SDB, and an interest in reducing wait times and costs have led to increasing interest in a TM-based approach for the management of SDB. This will become increasingly important as the Centers for Medicare and Medicaid Services shifts from a fee-for-service payment model toward a performance payment model based on Merit-Based Incentive Payment System (MIPS) and Advanced Alternative Payment Models (APMs) as part of the Medicare Access and CHIP Reauthorization Act of 2015 (MACRA). This chapter outlines a TM-based approach for the diagnosis and management of SDB and defines optimal patient populations for TM application.

Technical Considerations for Sleep Telemedicine

The AASM taskforce has provided guidelines on the proper implementation of TM in sleep [3]. These guidelines address synchronous, real-time provider patient interactions as well as asynchronous store-and-forward interactions such as HSAT monitoring and PAP machine data review.

The site of the patient's location is referred to as the "originating site" and the site of the provider's location is referred to as the "destination site or distant site." The equipment used should adhere to the guidelines put forth by the American Telemedicine Association [13, 14]. Sleep TM visits include synchronous live interactions and asynchronous interactions. Synchronous visits include live visits in real time, where the patient and the provider are separated by a distance and communicate via video conferencing. In essence, this functions as a live office visit and hence all technical standards, which would be adhered to in live office visits have to be met. Billing can be performed using Current Procedural Terminology (CPT) codes with a GT telehealth modifier.

Asynchronous visits are visits where the healthcare provider and the patient are separated by time in addition to distance. Care provided can include remote interpretation of data, electronic messaging, and self-care models.

Implementing sleep telemedicine requires the following essential elements [14, 15]:

- Presence of a remote monitoring device in the patient's home
- Means of electronically transmitting the data
- Encrypted storage of patient information to maintain patient confidentiality
- Feedback and advice provided to the patient through either live interaction with the healthcare provider or automated feedback based on a predetermined algorithm

Sleep TM visits are clinically beneficial, as well as cost- and time effective, when conducted for follow-up for sleep apnea patients on PAP therapy, in conjunction with review of PAP downloads. Such visits can troubleshoot PAP equipment and help to improve patient compliance with PAP therapy and can be conducted in the convenience of the patient's home.

Home-Based E-Evaluation of Sleep Disordered Breathing Via TM

Remote Healthcare Provider Evaluation

Clinical Video Telehealth (CVT) technology can be used effectively for evaluation and management of patients both with synchronous real-time provider-patient interaction as well as asynchronous interactions with review of PAP machine data via cloud-based platform such as Respironics Encoreanywhere [16] and ResMed Airview [17]. Healthcare systems such as Veterans Affairs Medical Centers (VAMC) have set up real-time clinic-based video telehealth systems that are being utilized at the author's institution for patients to have remote visits for management of SDB.

Sleep medicine can effectively use CVT as a significant portion of the diagnosis is clear from the history and physical examination, which can readily be carried out with a tele-stethoscope and a mobile camera at the originating site [3]. At the author's institution, patients present to Community-Based Outpatient Clinics (CBOC) that are distributed across the state. Patients are assisted by a patient services assistant (PSA) during the telehealth Sleep Medicine visit that is carried out remotely by the sleep physician based at the Portland VAMC. Patients have been receptive to the idea of sleep telehealth visits as reflected in survey studies by Bros and Kelly [11, 12]. In these two survey studies, 60–78% of individuals had a favorable response to telemonitoring of CPAP compliance suggesting that the idea of telemonitoring is acceptable to patients. A similar structure has been studied by VAMCs in Kansas City, Houston, and Philadelphia [7, 18, 19]. In all cases, the outcomes were similar between TM and in-person visits. In the study by Fields et al. dropout rates, CPAP adherence rates, and patient outcomes were similar between in-person and telemedicine visits at 3 months [7]. The study by Spaulding et al. showed that using telemedicine and intraoral camera, patient experience was very similar with telemedicine visits as an in-person visits (18).This approach has also been shown to work internationally in two published clinical trials from Spain [5, 20]. The studies evaluated both diagnosis of sleep apnea using HSAT as well as PAP delivery and compliance ensure that outcomes were similar in both in-person as well as telemedicine setting. In a recent study from Japan, telemedicine support for CPAP compliance, with monthly telemedicine follow-up and three monthly in-person visits improved adherence to CPAP from $45.8 \pm 18.2\%$ to $57.3 \pm 24.4\%$ [21]. This difference was statistically significant and similar to monthly in-person visits.

Based on the collective experiences of VAMCs as well as AASM guidelines [3], we recommend that institutions and centers focus on the following six steps to develop a sleep TM program:

1. Obtain buy-in from patients and providers regarding patient origination site and thus where patients would present for the remote visits for physician evaluation.
2. Budgeting and planning for remote personnel, CVT equipment, HSAT, and PAP supplies to meet payer standards (e.g., Medicare, Medicaid, and others).
3. Training of remote-site personnel for evaluation of patients, HSAT setup, PAP data download, and troubleshooting of devices.
4. Setting up robust telecommunications portal with appropriate bandwidth and backup systems including use of electronic health records at the originating and distant sites.
5. Procedures for management of inventory, HSAT equipment, and PAP supplies at the remote site.
6. Following up with remote site personnel and patients to evaluate satisfaction and to solve issues on a regular basis.

At our institution, providers perform key elements of sleep-relevant medical history as if it was an in-person visit and sleep diagnostics are performed in accordance with standards, clinical practice guidelines, and practice parameters established by AASM. PSAs work as patient presenters, facilitating communication between patients at the originating site and providers at the distant site. Primary care providers at the CBOCs, which act as the originating sites, help with patient evaluations and trained personnel help with PAP data download.

Home Sleep Testing for SDB

Home sleep apnea testing (HSAT) monitors are type three devices, which include at least four channels and must include at least two channels of respiratory movement or respiratory movement and airflow, one channel for heart rate or ECG, and one for oxygen saturation [22]. Electroencephalogram signals are usually not monitored, and hence sleep is not recorded. HSAT utilizes total recording time to generate a respiratory event index (REI) as opposed to traditional polysomnography, which uses total sleep time to generate an apnea-hypopnea index (AHI). For this reason, HSAT can have a high false-negative rate of up to 17% of patients for the detection of sleep apnea. Hence, high-risk individuals with a negative HSAT result should be followed up by an in-laboratory polysomnogram to definitely evaluate them for sleep apnea [23].

The American Academy of Sleep Medicine has recommended that HSAT should only be performed in conjunction with a comprehensive sleep evaluation, which in turn, should be performed by a board-certified sleep physician or a physician who has met the eligibility criteria for board certification in sleep medicine [23]. The indications and contraindications for HSAT are listed in Table 10.1.

Table 10.1 Indications and contraindications for home sleep apnea testing

Indications	Contraindications
High pretest probability of moderate to severe OSA	Not appropriate for screening of asymptomatic populations
Diagnoses of OSA in patients where a laboratory polysomnography is not possible	Presence of significant comorbidities: Moderate to severe pulmonary disease Neuromuscular disease Congestive heart failure
Monitor the response to non-CPAP treatment for OSA Oral appliances Upper airway surgery Weight loss	Presence of other sleep disorders: Central sleep apnea Periodic limb movement disorder Insomnia Parasomnia Circadian rhythm disorders Narcolepsy

Abbreviations: OSA obstructive sleep apnea, *CPAP* continuous positive airway pressure

A home-based approach for the diagnosis of SDB is an attractive concept as it can help to expedite diagnosis and treatment of populations with limited access to healthcare. The challenge of such an approach is ensuring acquisition of high quality data and adequate data transmission for interpretation by the treating provider. During a 24-month period, respiratory polygraphy (RP) was performed in 499 patients in 4 satellite outpatient clinics of a Buenos Aires hospital [24]. Four percent of the recordings were considered invalid and RP had to be repeated. Mild, moderate, and severe obstructive sleep apnea (OSA) was diagnosed in 33.5%, 22%, and 17.2% of the subjects, respectively. In this study, home-based testing for OSA with remote data transmission, manual scoring of data and clinical decision-making by pulmonologists, was found to be a reasonable strategy for the evaluation of suspected OSA in a high-risk population without significant comorbidities.

This underlines the importance of performing HSAT only in individuals with a moderate to high pre-test probability of OSA [25] without significant comorbidities.

Remote Follow-Up of Patients with SDB

PAP is highly efficacious for SDB treatment, but difficulty with adherence has limited its overall effectiveness [26–28]. A combination of PAP telemonitoring with automated feedback messaging improved 90-day compliance with PAP for SDB in a large 4 arm, randomized, factorial design clinical trial of 1455 patients in a large managed-care system [10]. The TM-based education when done alone improved clinic attendance but did not significantly change continuous positive airway pressure (CPAP) adherence [10].

Other studies have shown increased PAP adherence and associated improvement in patient outcomes with a TM-based approach [29, 30]. In a study from the Spanish Sleep Network, a TM-based strategy for the follow-up of patients on PAP treatment for SDB has been shown to be of comparable efficacy as standard hospital/clinic-based care for symptom improvement, PAP compliance, and to have comparable side effects and satisfaction rates [5]. In a study of TM-based management of OSA with HSAT, tele-medicine consultation, and auto-CPAP, patients in the TM group had similar outcomes with improved adherence to PAP as in the conventional consultation group [20]. Similarly, among CPAP-non-adherent patients, a nurse-led telehealth intervention demonstrated improvement in PAP adherence [30]. Studies at several VAMCs have also shown equal effectiveness of TM-based versus in-person programs for follow-up of patients with SDB and management of PAP therapy [4, 7]. These data suggest that a TM-based management program for SDB and PAP follow-up is a feasible and cost-effective approach with similar outcomes to conventional clinic follow-up programs.

The authors will provide here an outline of the program that is currently being used for patient evaluation and management at one of our institutions (Fig. 10.1). At the authors' institution, an electronic consult (e-consult) is placed by primary care

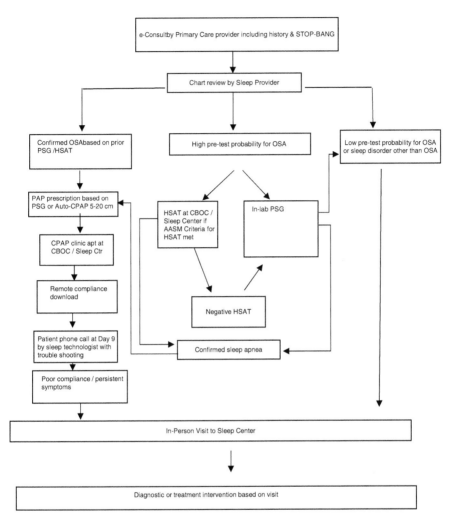

Fig. 10.1 Suggested algorithm for the management of patients with SDB incorporating a TM-based approach. *Abbreviations:* OSA obstructive sleep apnea, PSG polysomnography, HSAT home sleep apnea testing, CBOC Community-Based Outpatient Clinics, AASM American Academy of Sleep Medicine, CPAP continuous positive airway pressure

providers, which includes pertinent history and STOP-BANG questionnaire [31]. STOP-BANG questionnaire is a validated and widely used instrument for screening for OSA [32]. The sleep provider reviews the e-consult and patients who meet AASM criteria for HSAT [23] undergo HSAT at the Community Based Outreach Clinic. HSAT data are reviewed and if the patient has OSA and meets criteria, then the patient is provided with an Auto-CPAP set between 5 and 20 cm H2O. Data are downloaded remotely by a sleep technologist at 9 days and 30 days, and at each time point, the patient has a remote phone call with the technologist to troubleshoot CPAP issues.

Education about CPAP compliance is also provided. Patients with low pretest probability for OSA, those with symptoms of OSA and negative HSAT or in lab polysomnography or those who have poor CPAP compliance or persistent symptoms are provided an in-person visit to the sleep center. This approach has been studied in various settings and found to be as effective as the traditional care model [4, 5, 7, 19, 25].

Conclusion

Telemedicine has great utility in an era when OSA is becoming a very prevalent health concern and access to specialty expertise is limited due to a shortage of board-certified sleep physicians. TM in general, is well accepted by patients and can be used successfully in a large number of patients without significant comorbidities. It provides a more personalized approach to the management of OSA for each individual patient. Given the advantages of a TM-based approach, we expect it to assume a bigger role in the management of patients with OSA over time. Reimbursement for TM in the United States is gradually improving, which would lead to increased use of TM over time.

Future Directions

Current use of TM in sleep medicine is limited. There is tremendous potential to increase the use of TM in the management of SDB, given the cost-effectiveness, access to timely care, and improvement in PAP compliance seen with this approach. TM can help to facilitate long-term follow-up of patients with OSA who are on PAP devices. It can be used to provide one-on-one counseling to patients remotely, trouble shoot problems with PAP devices, and follow up the efficacy of PAP devices in OSA patients remotely. Other areas of development include use of smart phone applications for management of OSA. Evolving technology will further facilitate the role of TM in the diagnosis and management of SDB.

Declaration of Interest Dr. Lal has received grant support from Jazz Pharmaceuticals and Invado Pharmaceuticals and is a consultant for Jazz Pharmaceuticals, Cipla Pharmaceuticals, Suven Life Sciences, and Chest/GSK. Dr. Khan has received grant support from AstraZeneca, Glaxo Smith Cline, United Therapeutics, Actelion Pharmaceuticals, Reata Pharmaceuticals, and National Institutes of Health.

References

1. Peppard PE, Young T, Barnet JH, Palta M, Hagen EW, Hla KM. Increased prevalence of sleep-disordered breathing in adults. Am J Epidemiol. 2013;177(9):1006–14.

2. Watson NF, Rosen IM, Chervin RD. The past is prologue: the future of sleep medicine. J Clin Sleep Med. 2017;13(1):127–35.
3. Singh J, Badr MS, Diebert W, Epstein L, Hwang D, Karres V, et al. American Academy of Sleep Medicine (AASM) position paper for the use of telemedicine for the diagnosis and treatment of sleep disorders. J Clin Sleep Med. 2015;11(10):1187–98.
4. Baig MM, Antonescu-Turcu A, Ratarasarn K. Impact of sleep telemedicine protocol in management of sleep apnea: a 5-year VA experience. Telemed J E Health. 2016;22(5):458–62.
5. Isetta V, Negrin MA, Monasterio C, Masa JF, Feu N, Alvarez A, et al. A Bayesian cost-effectiveness analysis of a telemedicine-based strategy for the management of sleep apnoea: a multicentre randomised controlled trial. Thorax. 2015;70(11):1054–61.
6. Shin JC, Kim J, Grigsby-Toussaint D. Mobile phone interventions for sleep disorders and sleep quality: systematic review. JMIR Mhealth Uhealth. 2017;5(9):e131.
7. Fields BG, Behari PP, McCloskey S, True G, Richardson D, Thomasson A, et al. Remote ambulatory management of veterans with obstructive sleep apnea. Sleep. 2016;39(3):501–9.
8. Russo JE, McCool RR, Davies L. VA telemedicine: an analysis of cost and time savings. Telemed J E Health. 2016;22(3):209–15.
9. Hoet F, Libert W, Sanida C, Van den Broecke S, Bruyneel AV, Bruyneel M. Telemonitoring in continuous positive airway pressure-treated patients improves delay to first intervention and early compliance: a randomized trial. Sleep Med. 2017;39:77–83.
10. Hwang D, Chang JW, Benjafield AV, Crocker ME, Kelly C, Becker KA, et al. Effect of telemedicine education and telemonitoring on continuous positive airway pressure adherence. The tele-OSA randomized trial. Am J Respir Crit Care Med. 2018;197(1):117–26.
11. Bros JS, Poulet C, Arnol N, Deschaux C, Gandit M, Charavel M. Acceptance of telemonitoring among patients with obstructive sleep apnea syndrome: how is the perceived interest by and for patients? Telemed J E Health. 2017;24(5):351–9.
12. Kelly JM, Schwamm LH, Bianchi MT. Sleep telemedicine: a survey study of patient preferences. ISRN Neurol. 2012;2012:135329.
13. Gough F, Budhrani S, Cohn E, Dappen A, Leenknecht C, Lewis B, et al. ATA practice guidelines for live, on-demand primary and urgent care. Telemed J E Health. 2015;21(3):233–41.
14. Zia S, Sleep Telemedicine FBG. An emerging field's latest frontier. Chest. 2016;149(6):1556–65.
15. Goodridge D, Marciniuk D. Rural and remote care: overcoming the challenges of distance. Chron Respir Dis. 2016;13(2):192–203.
16. Smit M, Zuidhof AB, Bos SI, Maarsingh H, Gosens R, Zaagsma J, et al. Bronchoprotection by olodaterol is synergistically enhanced by tiotropium in a guinea pig model of allergic asthma. J Pharmacol Exp Ther. 2014;348(2):303–10.
17. Spina D. Pharmacology of novel treatments for COPD: are fixed dose combination LABA/LAMA synergistic? Eur Clin Respir J. 2015;2:26634.
18. Spaulding R, Stevens D, Velasquez SE. Experience with telehealth for sleep monitoring and sleep laboratory management. J Telemed Telecare. 2011;17(7):346–9.
19. Hirshkowitz M, Sharafkhaneh A. A telemedicine program for diagnosis and management of sleep-disordered breathing: the fast-track for sleep apnea tele-sleep program. Semin Respir Crit Care Med. 2014;35(5):560–70.
20. Coma-Del-Corral MJ, Alonso-Alvarez ML, Allende M, Cordero J, Ordax E, Masa F, et al. Reliability of telemedicine in the diagnosis and treatment of sleep apnea syndrome. Telemed J E Health. 2013;19(1):7–12.
21. Murase K, Tanizawa K, Minami T, Matsumoto T, Tachikawa R, Takahashi N, et al. A randomized controlled trial of telemedicine for long-term sleep apnea CPAP management. Ann Am Thorac Soc. 2019;17(3):329–37. https://doi.org/10.1513/AnnalsATS.201907-494OC.
22. Lux L, Boehlecke B, Lohr KN. Effectiveness of portable monitoring devices for diagnosing obstructive sleep apnea: update of a systematic review. Rockville: AHRQ Technology Assessments; 2004.
23. Collop NA, Anderson WM, Boehlecke B, Claman D, Goldberg R, Gottlieb DJ, et al. Clinical guidelines for the use of unattended portable monitors in the diagnosis of obstructive sleep

apnea in adult patients. Portable Monitoring Task Force of the American Academy of Sleep Medicine. J Clin Sleep Med. 2007;3(7):737–47.

24. Borsini E, Blanco M, Bosio M, Fernando DT, Ernst G, Salvado A. "Diagnosis of sleep apnea in network" respiratory polygraphy as a decentralization strategy. Sleep Sci. 2016;9(3):244–8.

25. Goldstein CA, Karnib H, Williams K, Virk Z, Shamim-Uzzaman A. The utility of home sleep apnea tests in patients with low versus high pre-test probability for moderate to severe OSA. Sleep Breath. 2018;22(3):641–51.

26. Sawyer AM, Gooneratne NS, Marcus CL, Ofer D, Richards KC, Weaver TE. A systematic review of CPAP adherence across age groups: clinical and empiric insights for developing CPAP adherence interventions. Sleep Med Rev. 2011;15(6):343–56.

27. Rotenberg BW, Murariu D, Pang KP. Trends in CPAP adherence over twenty years of data collection: a flattened curve. J Otolaryngol Head Neck Surg. 2016;45(1):43.

28. Marin JM, Carrizo SJ, Vicente E, Agusti AG. Long-term cardiovascular outcomes in men with obstructive sleep apnoea-hypopnoea with or without treatment with continuous positive airway pressure: an observational study. Lancet. 2005;365(9464):1046–53.

29. Sparrow D, Aloia M, Demolles DA, Gottlieb DJ. A telemedicine intervention to improve adherence to continuous positive airway pressure: a randomised controlled trial. Thorax. 2010;65(12):1061–6.

30. Smith CE, Dauz ER, Clements F, Puno FN, Cook D, Doolittle G, et al. Telehealth services to improve nonadherence: a placebo-controlled study. Telemed J E Health. 2006;12(3):289–96.

31. Chung F, Yegneswaran B, Liao P, Chung SA, Vairavanathan S, Islam S, et al. STOP questionnaire: a tool to screen patients for obstructive sleep apnea. Anesthesiology. 2008;108(5):812–21.

32. Nagappa M, Liao P, Wong J, Auckley D, Ramachandran SK, Memtsoudis S, et al. Validation of the STOP-bang questionnaire as a screening tool for obstructive sleep apnea among different populations: a systematic review and meta-analysis. PLoS One. 2015;10(12):e0143697.

Chapter 11
Telemedicine in the Practice of Emergency Medicine: Telemergency

Richard L. Summers, Sarah A. Sterling, and Danielle K. Block

Introduction

Rapid communication and consultation with advanced clinical specialists at the time of a medical emergency can potentially mean the difference between life and death. Telemedicine offers the promise of immediate connectivity to board-certified emergency physicians and other specialists in these acute circumstances. However, unlike other areas of telemedicine that focus on one type of specialty or medical condition, the broad nature of the practice of telemergency in the evaluation of the undifferentiated patient requires greater flexibility in engagement and has added challenges of timing and logistics. However, the growing volume of patients served and the great disparity in emergency care in many communities in the United States suggest that the use of telemedicine in the emergency department (ED) also presents a major opportunity for an impact on outcomes in the management of time-sensitive events.

What Is Telemergency?

A medical emergency is defined as an acute condition that without immediate intervention would result in the loss of life, limb, or a permanent disability. Almost every medical discipline from cardiology to dermatology has clinical scenarios in which such emergent interventions are required in a time-sensitive framework. While

R. L. Summers (✉) · S. A. Sterling
Department of Emergency Medicine, University of Mississippi Medical Center,
Jackson, MS, USA
e-mail: rsummers@umc.edu

D. K. Block
UMMC Center for Telehealth, University of Mississippi Medical Center, Jackson, MS, USA

© Springer Nature Switzerland AG 2021   161
D. W. Ford, S. R. Valenta (eds.), *Telemedicine*, Respiratory Medicine,
https://doi.org/10.1007/978-3-030-64050-7_11

emergency physicians are trained to recognize and stabilize most common emergency conditions, specialists with advanced expertise are sometimes required to provide additional definitive care (e.g., cesarean delivery for an acute placenta abruption). While the resources and spectrum of specialties that are available at most large urban EDs allow for the state-of-the-art management of most emergency conditions, the lack of such means in rural and smaller community hospitals presents a significant challenge when they are presented with acute medical conditions [1]. Telemergency is a process in which the disparities in expertise typically found in smaller hospital EDs can be ameliorated through the use of telemedicine technologies, a team of trained and supported advanced practice providers, and robust clinical resources at a "hub" site responsible for provision of telemergency [2]. The recommended general components, structure, and process of practice for such a telemergency system is outlined in Text Box 11.1 and based on more than 15 years of experience at the University of Mississippi Medical Center (UMMC).

Text Box 11.1 Telemergency Medicine Standards and Guidelines

A physician practicing telemergency in a Level I or Level II Trauma Center and functioning in a collaborative/consultative role shall observe the following protocols and standards:

- Emergency medicine physicians –the emergency medicine physician practicing telemergency medicine and functioning in a collaborative/consultative role should be board-certified in emergency medicine
- Hub site emergency medicine physician staffing – the emergency department of the level i or level ii trauma center (the "hub site") shall be continually staffed, 24 hours a day, 7 days a week, with board-certified emergency medicine physician(s). The telemergency program shall have a medical director who is board-certified in emergency medicine and shall serve as the director of the advanced practice provider training program.
- Hub site availability of specialists — the emergency medicine physician shall have access to the on-site specialists who are normally available at a level i trauma center. These specialists shall include, but not be limited to: neonatologists, pediatric intensivists, obstetricians, and trauma surgeons. They should be available for a consult within 30 minutes.
- It staff – the hub site shall be supported by information technology (it) specialists who are available to proactively monitor, address, and resolve technical issues at both the hub site and distant sites. Prior to the initiation of telemergency medicine, the medical director of the telemergency program shall review and approve a plan for prompt it responses to technology issues and problems. Any page shall be answered in less than 10 minutes and unless there is a network outage, the problem shall be resolved in less than 4 hours.
- Telestroke services – the hub site shall be staffed with emergency medicine physicians who meet the requirement stated above, and who are able and willing to assess for and recommend time-critical medications (e.g.,

Thrombolysis) when appropriate. Additionally, the hub site shall have immediate availability of stroke specialists.

- Transportation resources – the hub site shall maintain adequate resources to transport a patient from any distant site to the hub site within 60 minutes, or to transport an emergency medicine physician to the patient, if necessary.
- It hardware/software – the telemergency technology shall include telehealth equipment with high resolution capability, far end camera control and peripheral devices (stethoscope, otoscope, dermascope). Internet bandwidth shall be sufficient to have a seamless audio/video experience.
- Training program for advanced practice providers – the medical director at the hub site or the physician who serves as chief quality officer at the level i or level ii trauma center shall review and approve a formal training program for advanced practice providers who staff the distant partner sites. This will be a formalized course of training specific to the practice of telemergency medicine that includes simulation, skills and practical training, didactic training, and hands-on practical rotations at the hub site. Additionally, the training program will include an annual skills assessment of advanced practice providers for clinical procedures (suturing, intubation, chest tube placement, etc.)
- Continuous quality improvement – the hub site shall monitor and regularly analyze data to ensure continuous quality improvement and consistent outcomes in telemergency medicine.

Why Is There a Need for Telemedicine in Emergency Medicine?

According to the US Centers for Disease Control (CDC), there are approximately 136 million ED visits in the United States each year [3]. Of these visits almost 40 million are injury related (29%). Additionally, more than 12 million (9%) of the overall patients are hospitalized for protracted management, and of these, 1.5 million are admitted to intensive care units (ICUs). Around 2.2% of patient visits result in a transfer to a hospital with higher levels of care. Most of these transfers are from rural and smaller community hospitals.

To provide further context, an analysis of healthcare workforce needs reported that 20% of the US population resides in a rural setting, while only 9% of the physician workforce lives and works in these same areas and a majority of these are primary care practitioners [4]. For emergency care, Carr et al. found that living in a rural area is "a key variable in access to ED care," and noted profound association between rurality and overall access to emergent care [5]. Nationally it has been noted that the demand for board-certified emergency medicine (EM) trained physicians significantly exceeds the available supply [6]. So, as is the case with other specialists, rural hospitals struggle to recruit EM-trained physicians, with a large portion of ED care being provided by physicians trained in other specialties [7, 8]. In fact, the likelihood of receiving care from a board-certified emergency physician decreases fivefold as rurality increases [7, 8].

This is important because it has been demonstrated that both quality and timeliness of care with critical interventions is best achieved when emergency care is administered by EM board-certified physicians as compared to non-EM physicians [9–11]. The importance of this rural disparity is amplified when considering the numerous research studies that suggest that timely appropriate medical interventions are the critical determinant of outcomes in many emergent conditions such as ST-elevation myocardial infarctions (STEMI), traumatic shock, and acute ischemic stroke [12, 13]. Telemedicine support for non-specialist emergency providers practicing in rural and small community hospitals has been considered one potential pathway to improving the quality of emergency care in rural and underserved settings [2, 11].

History of Telemergency

The Telemergency Program at UMMC began as a pilot project with 3 hospitals in October 2003 [14]. The program was initially started with the assistance of private foundation funding acquired by Richard L. Summers, MD, and was conceptualized and organized by Robert L. Galli, MD, and Kristi Henderson, DNP, NP-BC [2, 14]. The program was born from a consensus within the UMMC Department of Emergency Medicine that there was a serious need to improve emergency care in Mississippi. At that time, UMMC frequently received poorly managed trauma and critical patients in transfer to our tertiary care ED from critical access hospitals in small rural communities where there were no physicians available with emergency expertise. Often these EDs were covered by local physicians who were also actively practicing in their clinics or they were being supported by nurse practitioners with a family medicine orientation. Recruiting board-certified EM physicians to cover these small EDs was financially unfeasible, but closure of these hospitals would place enormous burdens on their communities and require hours of travel to find the first available hospital for emergency services in already underserved population. Many other states confront similar issues.

We developed a strategy that combines EM-trained advanced practice providers and telemedicine connections to provide EM expertise to these struggling medical communities. Since 2003 the UMMC telemergency program has grown to include 17 rural hospital EDs and has serviced more than 600,000 patients in that 15-year period. With this system, we have assisted in leading cardiac resuscitations, delivering babies, and many other forms of acute care management in real time [11]. From this platform, we have launched air transport from the telemedicine consultation room for emergency transports and sent an emergency physician to distant sites in a time of disaster. We also support telemedicine sites on oil rigs in the Gulf of Mexico for emergent consultations. Since this initial program, similar successful models for telemergency have developed in other locations throughout the United States.

State of the Practice of Telemergency

The Telemergency Practice Model

A telemergency system functions as a virtual ED on a 24/7 basis with a board-certified EM physician stationed in the telemedicine operations center ready to answer all incoming requests [2]. Experience has taught us that the operations center should be contiguous with the Hub's ED to best allow for the utilization of additional resources and expertise when needed. Emergency consultations are typically available for any patient who arrives at one of the partner sites as determined by the provider at that location. However, minor conditions often do not require consultation and can be handled locally. A mutually acceptable protocol with consulting criteria can help guide this decision-making with a requirement for engagement with the telemergency consulting service for all higher acuity patients [15]. Such a triaged practice allows for the telemergency system to accommodate multiple EDs at the same time, while oversight is provided through consultation with an EM specialist. Ancillary technical and information technology (IT) support is also required 24/7 for a successful program. Access to the local electronic health record, electrocardiography, and radiology platforms are all important pieces of a telemergency program as this broader information is often needed for the consultation. Any prospective model of telemergency should be compliant with state laws and consistent with the policies of the state board of medical licensure. An example of standards that are commonly utilized is included at the end of this chapter.

Role for the Advanced Practice Provider

While telemergency consultation services can be provided to any ED that is not staffed with an EM physician, it is often found that supporting a qualified advanced practice provider offers the best utilization of resources in small rural communities with few emergency visits [16]. It has been our experience that a program that provides some specialty training in emergency skills such as intubations and chest tube placements enables confidence and integrity for the system. The scope of practice determined for these providers should be in agreement with the state's medical licensure boards for medicine and nursing.

Criteria for Telemergency Consultation

It is important to establish workflows and specific criteria for consultation in any tele-medicine system. The criteria currently used in our telemergency program at UMMC were developed over years of experience [2, 14, 16]. Initially, all patients were required to be treated and evaluated by both the advanced practice provider and the collaborating consultant EM physician through telemedicine. However, the experience of the program was that this comprehensive process was unwieldy in the evaluation of non-urgent patients and increased the wait time for minor complaints. We created a set of guidelines to identify specific patients whom the advanced practice providers could assess and treat primarily, as well as those patients requiring immediate consultation and transfer. These detailed guidelines are provided in Tables 11.1, 11.2, and 11.3 and are divided into 3 categories: (1) does not require consultation, (2) does require consultation, and (3) does require consultation and probable transfer. These categories are based on decision points of emergencies needing advanced expertise and also the potential need for transfer. While these guidelines serve as a baseline for telemergency consultation, they may not precisely cover every situation and clinical venue. Further research is needed to assess the risks and benefits of such guidelines and their implementation as well as potential adaptations to meet needs in other clinical contexts.

Telemedicine Equipment

Telemedicine equipment mounted on a mobile cart allows for two-way audio and visual communication between the patient or distant provider and the EM physician in the ED-based operations center. The technology allows for a remote, yet thorough exam including peripheral devices that enable the ability to auscultate the heart and lungs, and to examine the inner ear, nose, and skin. Technology can be utilized to complete any portion of the exams as if in-person except for those involving smell and touch. There are also mechanisms in place for the electronic downloading and surveillance of radio-graphic images, laboratory data, and electrocardiograms from the distant site.

Telemergency Business Models

The need for sustainable business models is pervasive in telehealth. For telemer-gency, there are two common business models that can achieve this goal: contractual services or fee-for-service. Presently, the simplest approach is to provide the service under a contractual arrangement with the hospital receiving telemergency services. Such an agreement could provide for a prespecified fee assessed for each documented tele-encounter or be a global charge for coverage on an hourly/daily/monthly basis. In our experience, a global charge approach is preferable since it empowers rural providers to have a low threshold for requesting a consult and

Table 11.1 Conditions that do not require telemergency consultation

Abdominal pain: stable vitals, no significant physical examination findings, age < 50 years
Allergic reactions not associated with shortness of breath, wheezing, or hypotension
Animal bites not involving the hand or face
Cerumen removal
Chronic peripheral vascular disease
Conjunctivitis
Constipation/diarrhea
Contact dermatitis
Dental pain
Dizziness: vital signs stable, no significant physical examination findings, age < 50 years
Fatigue without associated symptoms
Follow-up wound check, cast check, or suture removal
Foreign body removal (uncomplicated and not involving the eye)
Gastritis: suspected food poisoning, no associated dehydration with limited duration
Gynecologic disorders: vaginitis, insignificant abnormalities in menstruation, cramps
Hemorrhoids
Hypertension that is asymptomatic and accompanied by a diastolic pressure < 120 mm Hg
Incision and drainage of simple abscess not involving rectal area
Intravenous hydration/antibiotics >8 years old
Low back pain that is chronic and not associated with neurologic findings
Migraines: typical migraine, stable vital signs, afebrile, normal examination, no trauma
Minor burns
Minor eye injury: corneal abrasion
Minor lacerations or abrasions
Nausea/vomiting
Otitis media, otitis externa, ear pain >3 months old
Pharyngitis: no sign of abscess or airway compromise
Pregnancy without bleeding, pain
Prescription refills: non-narcotic or controlled substance until next business day
Puncture wounds not requiring exploration
Sexually transmitted diseases, excluding pelvic inflammatory disease
Skin rashes, pruritus
Sprains/strains
Swollen lymph nodes
Uncomplicated hepatitis or exposure to hepatitis
Upper respiratory infection, congestion, cough, flu
Urinary tract infections >6 months old
Work releases
Wound care
Any of the above conditions with the presence of a complex medical history or at the discretion of the nurse practitioner may require consultation.

Table 11.2 Conditions that require telemergency consultation

Abdominal pain: all patients with acute pain or >50 years old
Abnormal vital signs: SBP < 100 or >180 mm Hg, pulse rate <50 or >110 bpm, RR > 24 bpm, temperature >101.5 °F
Age <1 or >75 years (all patients)
Alcohol or drug withdrawals
Allergic reaction with shortness of breath, wheezing, or hypotension
Arrhythmias
Bleeding: significant bleeding from any orifice
Burns: any 3°; 2° >10% BSA; burns to face, hands, feet, perineum, electrical or inhalation
Chest pain: all patients
Coma or change in mental status
Complicated lacerations
Drug overdose
Fever, <6 months old
Fever and toxic appearance or of unknown origin, < 1 year old
Foreign body of the eye
Fractures with vascular impairment or displacement
Significant head trauma
Headache associated with neurologic findings, fever, or meningeal signs
Hypothermia, temperature <35 °C (95 °F); hyperthermia, temperature >40.5 °C (105 °F)
Hypertension: diastolic blood pressure of >120 mm Hg
Intravenous hydration/antibiotics in children <8 years old
Neurologic deficits
Severe pain management
Patient with complex medical history
Pelvic inflammatory disease
Postoperative-related problems
Postpartum pelvic pain
Pregnancy complications (i.e., abdominal pain, bleeding, fever)
Psychiatric patients with abnormal findings
Puncture wounds requiring exploration
Seizures
Shock
Shortness of breath
Sickle cell crisis
Testicular pain
Upper abdominal pain not clearly of gastrointestinal origin (possible cardiac)
Urinary tract infection/dysuria/hematuria in children <4 months old
Vaginal bleeding: saturation of full-size pad 1 or more per 2 hour
Any symptom that the provider is concerned about requires consultation
Any patient with the following laboratory tests ordered requires consultation:
EKG, computed tomography scan, cardiac enzymes, lumbar puncture, cervical-spine X-rays.

SBP systolic blood pressure, *bpm* beats per minute, *BSA* body surface area, *EKG* electrocardiogram

Table 11.3 Conditions that require telemergency consultation and probable transfer

Acute head injury
Advanced airway management: intubation
All resuscitations
Burn management
Dizziness with unstable vital signs
Multisystem trauma evaluation and resuscitation
Serious or complex medical emergencies (i.e., DKA)
Shock of any cause
Transfer of these patients should not be delayed because of the telemedicine consultation, but these consults should be used for the stabilization of these patients. Definitive treatment of these patients should not occur in the outlying emergency departments. Referral should be made to the closest appropriate facility capable of providing the services needed.

DKA diabetic ketoacidosis

mitigates the risk of missing patients who might benefit from telemergency consultation. The global model is also consistent with numerous medical professional contracts for conventional care in which the consultant is paid for "on call" time, thus ensuring availability even without utilization.

As healthcare systems grow and evolve, telehealth has become increasingly mainstream. Thus, third-party payers often reimburse for telehealth services, albeit with substantial variation at the state level and across commercial insurers. An important future direction is educating third-party payers with regard to the potential improvements in quality and cost associated with a telemergency program. Research regarding the changes in ED length of stay, tests ordered, transfers to other facilities, and general outcomes resulting from telemergency consultations will be important in providing evidence to obtain third-party payers' support.

Specific Clinical Scenarios and Telemergency

While telemergency services are intended to be broad and encompass all potential emergent conditions, there are at least four clinical contexts in emergency care that warrant further consideration. Sometimes an area of specialty expertise is needed that is beyond the typical scope of the consulting EM physician. Layering these specialty services on the backbone of a robust telemergency system is a practical solution to optimize certain specialty consults.

Telestroke

Treatment with thrombolytic therapy for the treatment of nonhemorrhagic acute stroke events substantially improves patient outcomes, and thus this emergency practice is standard of care in neurology. However, a national shortage of neurologists has placed a strain on the stroke specialists providing oversight for this evaluation and treatment on a 24/7 basis. Since most acute stroke patients first present to an ED, there is a compounded burden placed on facilities where neurologists are not readily available to provide for management oversight. Telestroke programs in which a neurologist can remotely consult with underserved EDs through telemedicine technologies have become a mainstream solution [17]. However, the stroke neurology workforce is quickly becoming overwhelmed with the variety of potential stroke candidates and stroke mimics that are identified by the nonemergency personnel for neurology consultation in the rural and small community hospitals. A hybrid system integrates telestroke services on the backbone of an established telemergency program in which EM physician specialists first triage the patients from the perspective of an undifferentiated emergency and then connect the partner site to a stroke specialist video-conferenced into the telemedicine consultation when appropriate [18].

Telepsychiatry

Mental health services are currently in great demand throughout the United States. Because of inadequate access to mental health services, many mentally ill patients seek care in EDs. Telepsychiatry expertise in the assessment of these patients before transfer to an acute care setting can greatly facilitate the disposition of these patients and significantly reduce overutilization of acute care systems. Therefore, telepsychiatry is becoming one of the most important aspects of a telemergency system. While the telemergency specialists can provide for a triage with metabolic and toxicology screening for these patients, the system that has access to further input by psychiatric specialists has significant advantages for initial mental health stabilization and triage decision making among this vulnerable patient population.

Teletrauma

It is usually considered that rural communities experience proportionately similar amounts of trauma as urban centers though the types of trauma may differ. However, because the populations of these communities are so small, the total number of trauma patients coming to rural EDs is much less than that seen in urban centers [19]. As with any area of medical practice, a reduced number of overall trauma encounters limits the experience of these ED personnel in dealing with certain types of severe injuries. It is thought that a telemedicine-assisted evaluation of trauma patients provides for a more comprehensive assessment and management of these patients and facilitates early transfers [13]. This is particularly important for the most severely injured patients with time-sensitive conditions requiring surgical and/ or specialty interventions.

The implementation of telemergency services in rural EDs in Mississippi was found by Duchesne et al. to improve the initial trauma evaluation and provide for more rapid transfer of severely injured patients to the trauma center [13]. This resulted in a significant overall reduction in mortality. Total hospital costs and lengths of stay were also reduced in this process. An analysis of trauma registry patients in North Dakota demonstrated decreases in length of ED stay for transferred trauma patients, with an implication of improved evaluations for those patients who were not transferred. However, this analysis noted that there was not an overall decrease in the transfer rate for trauma patients from the rural hospitals in which telemedicine was being utilized. This is not unexpected as it is usually the most severely injured patients who are transferred regardless of the capacity for evaluation by the local ED and due to lack of available advanced specialty services such as orthopedics or plastic surgery in rural settings. Perhaps the greatest benefit of connectivity to a telemergency system for trauma and other time-sensitive conditions is that if helicopter or other transfer transport is required, there is more immediate access to the Level I facility for acceptance of the patient and making the transfer arrangement.

Critical Care Support Through Telemedicine

Timely, quality care in life-threatening conditions is particularly challenging in rural areas due to the lack of specialty services and advanced experience in managing critical illness (Sterling SA. Critical Care Utilization in TelEmergency. Society of Academic Emergency Medicine abstract: in submission.) This consideration has been a major driver for the adoption of telemergency services among rural hospitals. A standardized approach to guiding any engagement with specialists through telemergency (as outlined in Tables 11.1, 11.2, and 11.3) is important to providing safe quality care.

In a recent analysis of 3946 consults in a mature telemergency program, 13.5% of the consults had ≥1 critical care diagnoses [20]. The top four critical care diagnoses were as follows: significant traumatic injury (16.9%), cardiopulmonary arrest (CPA 15.8%), myocardial infarction (15.6%), and cerebrovascular accident (10.9%). An inter-hospital occurred for 79.3% of the telemergency consults, with the outcome of death in the ED in 12.6% of the cases. Transfer hospital data show a median transfer distance of 62.3 miles with an estimated transfer time of 60 minutes by ground transport. These data support the implicit need for telemergency services among rural hospitals.

With regard to CPA specifically, a recent report by Summers et al. compared survival between urban patients with CPA managed via standard ED code teams and those in rural hospitals managed via telemedicine, and found no statistically significant difference between the groups. Of the 459 urban patient records examined, 114 patients survived (24.8%) CPA as compared to the 8 of 39 total rural patients (20.5%) [21]. These findings suggest that resuscitation guided by telemedicine consultation with emergency specialists can achieve survival rates among rural patients with CPA comparable to those of urban hospitals. Thus, narrowing the gap between the level of care found in rural and urban hospitals should be a major goal of any telemergency program.

EMS and Telemedicine

There are a variety of innovative possibilities for using telemedicine technologies in the prehospital setting [22]. As concerns for early differentiation, emergent treatment and appropriate routing of patients become more important for conditions such as stroke and trauma, a deeper engagement of EMS personnel with emergency experts will be important. In rural settings, the transport of critical individuals to advanced care centers may take longer than the typical "golden hour" considered for these patients [23]. Audiovisual and other electronic connectivity of telemergency support services to ambulances may provide life-saving decision support.

Epidemics, Bioterrorism, and Disaster Telemedicine

Emergent public health epidemics and bioterrorism attacks may first appear as sentinel events in the ED environments. Syndromic biosurveillance attached to telemergency services can provide a means for the early detection and response to these events [24]. In times of a major disaster, it is also often difficult to provide timely specialty expertise to the scene of the event [25]. Telemergency support has already been found to be useful in our program during disaster circumstances such as post-natural disaster medical support (e.g., hurricane and tornado) and during a Gulf of Mexico oil spill disaster. We may also see the future implementation of drone and GPS technologies in prehospital settings to support the response to telemergency disaster management.

Future of Telemergency

The future of telemedicine in general is one of rapid growth and dramatic changes in the landscape of healthcare enabled by significant advances in technology. There are many possibilities surrounding augmented reality instruments, remote-controlled robots, drones, and numerous other emerging technologies. Augmented reality is the use of computer-generated perceptual information in an immersive interactive experience in order to enhance the conditions and components of the real-world environment. The interactions can occur across multiple sensory modalities and could include visual, auditory, haptic, somatosensory, and olfactory experiences. Since a large part of the practice of medicine includes the skill of the physical examination, platforms that augment the telemedicine experience can provide valuable additional sensory information regarding the patient's condition to the teleprovider. For instance, if the emergency physician or surgeon providing the telemergency service can virtually palpate the abdomen through augmented technology to determine the characteristics of relative rigidity and tenderness, this may enable better management decisions and resultant impacts on triage decisions and related outcomes. Augmented reality technologies are rapidly being developed for military and entertainment uses. There is an expectation that they will also find uses in the practice of telemedicine. Since medical emergencies require time-sensitive decision-making, these innovations may find their greatest impact in the arena of telemergency.

Research in Telemergency

Telemedicine will likely be key to the survival of the rural and small community practice of EM. While we can make intuitive conclusions concerning the impact of these changes on patient outcomes, objective research will be critically important to validate the methods and practice of telemedicine. The two greatest challenges to doing robust outcomes-based research in telemergency are the episodic nature of the ED patient-physician relationship and the problems associated with complete data capture for the encounter across two distinct and distant locations [26]. The nearly ubiquitous utilization of electronic health records and the development of statewide health information exchange networks will greatly facilitate patient encounter data capture in the future.

Operational Metrics

Additional evidence supporting the value of the practice of telemergency on ED and hospital operational metrics continues to emerge. An analysis of data from our telemergency systems has demonstrated significant 20.1% increase in inpatient admissions locally at the rural facility and a 10.9% increase in appropriate patient transfers to a hospital with a higher level of care or specialty care unavailable at the rural hospital [11, 27]. The median change in death prevalence rates decreased 3.7% ($p = 0.88$), and there was a significant decrease in the prevalence rate of those who left without treatment (LWT) or left against medical advice (AMA) after a telemergency program implementation.

An evaluation of the routine use of the telemedicine system revealed that more than 54% of the rural providers used the telemedicine system for an audio/visual consultation every shift and more than 91% collaborated with the telemergency physician multiple times during their shift. This constant physician availability through telemedicine increased the frequency of consultations by 86.4% during the evaluation period. The nurse practitioners were comfortable with the use of the equipment (100%), and all were satisfied or very satisfied with the telemergency program. Operational and satisfaction metrics are important for the continued support of telemergency programs and should be routinely tracked.

Teleconsenting

The ED is often a point of recruitment for clinical research studies [28]. Teleconsenting allows a researcher to remotely video conference with a potential study participant and guide them through the informed consent document, going step-by-step until all required documentation is complete. Although teleconsenting is not meant to be used as the sole mode of enrollment for studies, it is a useful tool in a clinical researcher's recruitment arsenal, and can help overcome difficulties in meeting study number enrollment and diversity goals, particularly in rare disease cohorts. With the advent of new technology including free, secure sites such as doxy.me and the vast majority of US adults (77%) now owning smartphones, teleconsenting can take place in some of the most geographically remote locations such as rural EDs, saving researchers' time, decreasing study costs, and bringing forth valuable scientific developments more rapidly. Randomized, controlled trials show that participants are just as satisfied, in some cases more so, with the experience of teleconsenting, and have practically identical levels of research consent comprehension compared to standard face-to-face consenting [28, 29]. Teleconsenting will help advance research by increasing the potential reach of researchers without increasing costs, thereby aiding in recruitment and increasing inclusivity, diversity, and study power, while conserving regulatory requirements and participant satisfaction and comprehension.

References

1. Macy J Jr. The role of emergency medicine in the future of American medical care. Ann Emerg Med. 1995;25(2):230–3.
2. Galli R, Keith JC, McKenzie K, Hall GS, Henderson K. TelEmergency: a novel system for delivering emergency care to rural hospitals. Ann Emerg Med. 2008;51(3):275–84.
3. National Center for Health Statistics. FastStats: Emergency Department visits. Centers for Disease Control and Prevention. https://www.cdc.gov/nchs/fastats/emergency-department.htm
4. van Dis J. Where we live: health care in rural vs urban America. JAMA. 2002;287(1):108.
5. Carr BG, Branas CC, Metlay JP, Sullivan AF, Camargo CA Jr. Access to emergency care in the United States. Ann Emerg Med. 2009;54(2):261–9.
6. Sullivan AF, Ginde AA, Espinola JA, Camargo CA Jr. Supply and demand of board-certified emergency physicians by U. S. State, 2005. Acad Emerg Med. 2009;16:1014–8.
7. Groth H, House H, Overton R, Deroo E. Board-certified emergency physicians comprise a minority of the emergency department workforce in Iowa. West J Emerg Med. 2013;14:186–90.

8. Peterson LE, Dodoo M, Bennett KJ, Bazemore A, Phillips RL Jr. Nonemergency medicine-trained physician coverage in rural emergency departments. J Rural Health. 2008;24(2):183–8.
9. McNamara RM, Kelly JJ. Impact of an emergency medicine residency program on the quality of care in an urban community hospital emergency department. Ann Emerg Med. 1992;21(5):528–33.
10. Jones JH, Weaver CS, Rusyniak DE, Brizendine EJ, McGrath RB. Impact of emergency medicine faculty and an airway protocol on airway management. Acad Emerg Med. 2002;9:1452–6.
11. Sterling SA, Seals SR, Jones AE, King MH, Galli RL, Isom KC, et al. The impact of the TelEmergency program on rural emergency care: an implementation study. J Telemed Telecare. 2017;23:588–94.
12. Weaver CS, Avery SJ, Brizendine EJ, McGrath RB. Impact of emergency medicine faculty on door to thrombolytic time. J Emerg Med. 2004;26(3):279–83.
13. Duchesne JC, Kyle A, Simmons J, Islam S, Schmieg RE Jr, Olivier J, McSwain NE Jr. Impact of telemedicine upon rural trauma care. J Trauma. 2008;64:92–7.
14. Summers RL, Henderson K, Isom KC, Galli RL. The anniversary of TelEmergency. J Miss State Med Assoc. 2013;54(12):340–1.
15. Ward MM, Ullrich F, Mackinney AC, Bell AL, Shipp S, Mueller KJ. Tele-emergency utilization: in what clinical situations is tele-emergency activated? J Telemed Telecare. 2016;22:25–31.
16. Henderson K. TelEmergency: distance emergency care in rural emergency departments using nurse practitioners. J Emerg Nurs. 2006;32(5):388–93.
17. Zhai YK, Zhu WJ, Hou HL, Sun DX, Zhao J. Efficacy of telemedicine for thrombolytic therapy in acute ischemic stroke: a meta-analysis. J Telemed Telecare. 2015;21(3):123–30.
18. Isom KC, Summers RL, Henderson K. Integration of Telestroke services into an established telemedicine system. International Stroke Conference. Stroke. 2014;45:AWP294.
19. Hsia R, Shen YC. Possible geographical barriers to trauma center access for vulnerable patients in the United States: an analysis of urban and rural communities. Arch Surg. 2011;146:46–52.
20. Dharmar M, Romano PS, Kuppermann N, Nesbitt TS, Cole SL, Andrada ER, et al. Impact of critical care telemedicine consultations on children in rural emergency departments. Crit Care Med. 2013;41:2388–95.
21. Henderson K, Woodward LH, Isom KC, Summers RL. Relative survivability of cardiopulmonary arrest in rural emergency departments utilizing telemedicine. J Rural Emerg Med. 2014;1(1):9–12.
22. Galli R. Innovation possibilities for prehospital providers. Prehosp Emerg Care. 2006;10(3):317–9.
23. Newgard CD, Meier EN, Bulger EM, Buick J, Sheehan K, Lin S, et al. Revisiting the "Golden hour": an evaluation of out-of-hospital time in shock and traumatic brain injury. Ann Emerg Med. 2015;66(1):30–41.
24. Kemp AM, Clark MS, Dobbs T, Galli R, Sherman J, Cox R. Top 10 facts you need to know about synthetic cannabinoids: not so nice spice. Am J Med. 2016;129(3):240–4.
25. Carenzo L, Barra FL, Ingrassia PL, Colombo D, Costa A, Della Corte F. Disaster medicine through Google Glass. Eur J Emerg Med. 2015;22(3):222–5.
26. Dharmar M, Kuppermann N, Romano PS, Yang NH, Nesbitt TS, Phan J, et al. Telemedicine consultations and medication errors in rural emergency departments. Pediatrics. 2013;132:1090–7.
27. Sterling SA, Novotny NR, Puskarich MA, McKenzie LK, Summers RL, Jones AE. Consults in TelEmergency: a descriptive analysis. J Miss State Med Assoc. 2019;LX(3):111–4.
28. Bobb MR, Van Heukelom PG, Faine BA, Ahmed A, Messerly JT, Bell G, Mohr NM. Telemedicine provides non-inferior research informed consent for remote study enrollment: a randomized controlled trial. Acad Emerg Med. 2016;23(7):759–65.
29. Welch BM, Marshall E, Qanungo S, Aziz A, Laken M, Lenert L, Obeid J. Teleconsent: a novel approach to obtain informed consent for research. Contemp Clinl Trials Commun. 2016;3:74–9.

Chapter 12
Tele-ICU Programs

Daniel M. Hynes, Isabelle Kopec, and Nandita R. Nadig

Introduction

The changing demographics of the population in the United States are creating new challenges for healthcare providers. Americans are living longer with more complicated medical comorbidities [1, 2]. This, along with increased emphasis to deliver effective, expert-level care, has increased the need for critical care services [1, 3]. One major challenge in meeting these needs is a national shortage of intensivists estimated in a 2006 Health Resources and Services Administration (HRSA) study to be more than 1500 critical care specialists by 2020. These deficits are more pronounced in rural areas [4] where 25% of the US population resides, but which have only 10% of US physicians [5]. For critical care services, intensivist-directed care in an intensive care unit (ICU) has been shown to improve mortality, reduce ICU length of stay, and lower cost of care among critically ill patients [2, 6–8]. Currently, only 14% of patients admitted to ICUs receive intensivist-directed care, despite best practice recommendations that all ICU beds have such oversight [1, 8].

Intensivist-directed care models, sometimes termed "closed ICUs" tend to be at large health systems with deeper resources and greater economies of scale. Smaller, rural hospitals with limited resources are less likely to be able to achieve intensivist-directed oversight for their ICU patients [3, 9]. Thus, ICU telehealth was developed to bridge the gap between the need for expert-level critical care oversight to a larger proportion of the US population than can be achieved through conventional care

D. M. Hynes
Department of Pulmonary, Critical Care, Allergy, and Sleep Medicine, Medical University of South Carolina, Charleston, SC, USA

I. Kopec
Department of Critical Care, Advanced ICU Care, Creve Coeur, MO, USA

N. R. Nadig (✉)
Department of Medicine, Medical University of South Carolina, Charleston, SC, USA
e-mail: nadig@musc.edu

© Springer Nature Switzerland AG 2021
D. W. Ford, S. R. Valenta (eds.), *Telemedicine*, Respiratory Medicine,
https://doi.org/10.1007/978-3-030-64050-7_12

177

delivery models [8, 9]. From a centralized operations center, an inter professional team of critical care providers can offer numerous services to ICU patients in multiple remote locations simultaneously and based on real-time patient needs [3].

Telehealth is a broadly inclusive term for medical services delivered from a remote location using audiovisual communication technologies [1, 10]. In the 1990s, the robust expansion of computer and Internet technology capabilities began to enable telehealth as a viable form of healthcare delivery [11]. One of the first and most enduring successes of telehealth for a critically ill patient population was for the recognition and treatment of acute cerebrovascular accidents. First reported in 1999, multiple studies have validated the practicality and efficacy of audiovisual technology to provide emergent consultation with stroke experts for providers in areas that otherwise would not have access to these services [12–14].

In this same time period, telehealth started being utilized in the ICU. ICU telehealth is the delivery of care for critically ill patients by an intensivist from a remote location using electronic transfer of information through interactive audiovisual tools [10, 15]. While telestroke provides individual, as-needed consultative interactions, ICU telehealth is traditionally grounded in the telehealth paradigm of continuous remote patient monitoring [8, 11] that includes longitudinal, continual support for patients and providers. This can include tracking vital sign trends, lab monitoring, radiograph interpretation, reviewing archived data and notes, responding to alarms, and assisting in decision-making for on-site providers [1]. For purposes of this chapter, the term "teleICU" refers to the continuous remote patient monitoring teleICU model and not the consultative/episodic ICU telehealth model, unless otherwise identified.

The first demonstration-of-concept study was in a single surgical ICU at Johns Hopkins Hospital in 1997 [3]. This before-after study demonstrated decreased severity-adjusted ICU mortality (range of 46–68%), severity-adjusted hospital mortality (range of 30–33%), complications (range of 44–50%), and cost (range from 33–36%) [16]. A similar report was derived from Sentara Hospital in Norfolk, Virginia, in 2000, which also demonstrated reduced severity-adjusted ICU and hospital mortality of 60% and 30%, respectively [1]. These results were attributed to higher rates of adherence to best practice policies and improved response time to alerts and alarms for physiologic instability associated with teleICU [9].

Despite comparatively weak study designs, these initial reports of improvements in mortality, costs, and length of stay (LOS) sparked a surge in technology development and implementation of teleICU programs around 2003 [9]. It also led to the commercialization of remote monitoring technologies and services [3, 8]. Subsequently teleICU growth has been exponential with the addition of approximately 50 programs at 250 hospitals when last evaluated by the New England Health Care Institute (NEHI) and the Massachusetts Technology Collaborative 2010 report [17]. This rapid growth was attributed to adopter hospitals embracing teleICU for enhanced patient safety, improved outcomes through standardization of care, reduction in preventable complications, increased access to expertise, and mitigating the workforce shortage in critical care [3, 18, 19]. Subsequently, 30 major teleICU commercial vendors in the United States have found a niche market

[8]. Given the broad range of technologies and vendors available for consultative/episodic ICU telehealth, current prevalence reports of teleICU may be an under representation.

Kahn et al. performed a retrospective study of hospital characteristics using Centers for Medicare and Medicaid Services (CMS) from 2003 to 2010 to analyze the adoption of teleICU programs across the country [20]. In 2003, only 16 hospitals (0.4% of all hospitals included in the cohort) utilized teleICU, but at study termination in 2010, 213 hospitals (4.6%) had implemented teleICU programs. Interestingly, the rate of ICU bed coverage increased 101% in the first 4 years of the study, but then markedly slowed to 8.1% over the last 4 years. The rapid rise in ICU bed coverage seen earlier in the study was attributed to the aforementioned early studies demonstrating reduced mortality and cost, as well as the development of commercial teleICU programs in 2000 [1, 16, 20]. The authors hypothesized that the sharp reduction in growth was due to technology reaching a saturation point, and that the major barriers of cost and lack of reimbursement would prevent further implementation [20]. Four years later, however, Lilly et al. [1] reported ICU telehealth covered 11% of all ICU beds, with an expected growth rate of 1% per year. The same study also suggested that the critical care delivery models utilizing teleICU will surpass bedside intensivist programs in the future [1]. A recent review article by Vranas et al. corroborates this expected rate of teleICU increase at 15% usage in 2018 [7]. With the requirement of electronic medical records and computerized physician order entry mandated under the Affordable Care Act, it is reasonable to expect that medical services will continue to be digitalized and increase the opportunities for the growth of telehealth in the ICU setting.

Characteristics of Tele-ICU Programs

ICU telehealth programs are capable of providing a wide variety of support services to receiving organizations. The general responsibilities of the teleICU team will include trending physiologic variables such as vital signs and labs to prevent or identify earlier clinical deterioration, review imaging, respond to alarms, assess patients via cameras, provide oversight during crises, and oversee and carry out the comprehensive daily plans established by the local, onsite ICU team [2, 3, 8]. TeleICU providers utilize local electronic health records, computer order entry, telemetry, imaging software, as well as risk-prediction algorithms embedded into a central dashboard that can activate push notifications to accomplish these tasks [2, 8]. In addition to these direct clinical responsibilities, the teleICU program should develop high-quality informatics systems that allow for auditing, benchmarking, and compliance checks as elaborated on below [8, 21].

The teleICU team composition can be variable. In general, the team will consist of board-certified intensivists, critical care nurses, and advanced practitioners. Additional providers, such as respiratory therapists, pharmacists, and data specialists, may also be incorporated into the team [8]. The size and composition of the team depends on the number of ICU beds that require coverage. A smaller network, which is typically fewer than 70 beds, is usually staffed by 1 intensivist and 1 critical care nurse [8]. Additional nurses are typically added above 70 beds, and additional physicians are usually required when covering more than 120 beds [8]. The overall goal is not to take autonomy away from the bedside team but to improve safety and enhance outcomes through standardization and collaboration with the bedside ICU team [21].

To optimize teleICU resources and fully leverage its potential, designing and implementing a program should be a collaborative effort between the remote teleICU group and the regional facility providing patient care at the bedside. A fundamental step in implementation is first establishing the needs of the receiving institution. The intensity of the teleICU interaction care can be customized based on time, reactivity, and scope to meet these needs [7]. The overall goal is to utilize remote intensivists to provide uninterrupted critical care oversight at all times [8]. For example, a continuous, 24-7 teleICU coverage model may be needed if no intensivist is on staff at a hospital and ICUs are staffed by non-critical care-trained physicians. Alternatively, intermittent tele-ICU coverage can be instituted as needed when the local intensivist is in clinic, or no nocturnal or weekend coverage is available [8].

The coverage provided by the tele-ICU team may be proactive, reactive, scheduled, or some combination of all three. In the proactive model, tele-ICU intensivists provide continuous tracking of patient data trends to try and intervene before clinical deterioration occurs. This model will prompt periodic completion of tasks such as best practice compliance audits, and review of labs and imaging [8]. In a reactive model, tele-ICU intensivists respond to unscheduled requests, often urgent, from bedside providers or to automated tasks generated by a central dashboard. In a scheduled intervention model, the remote tele-ICU team will check in with the bedside team at specified intervals such as shift changes or for specific clinical activities such as weaning from mechanical ventilation [7]. These care delivery activities are not mutually exclusive and are typically combined to optimize meeting the needs of the patient and bedside ICU team [7].

The scope of involvement and autonomy of the tele-ICU team can vary and should be clearly specified at program inception. Some institutions will authorize tele-ICU intensivists to function as completely autonomous providers, capable of ordering medications, changing ventilator parameters, providing code team leadership, changing treatment plans, and participating in goals of care discussions. In fact, some teams incorporate tele-ICU providers into daily multidisciplinary rounds to obtain expert insight while formulating daily patient treatment plans [6, 7]. Alternatively, receiving hospital protocols and/or primary physicians may limit the power of the tele-ICU providers to the point where they may only respond to emergencies, and do not have authority to order routine medications and change treatment plans [7]. The scope of practice of the tele-ICU group may exist on a spectrum between these two extremes. To best optimize the clinical utility of a tele-ICU program, there should be a clear transition of care between remote care teams and bedside providers to ensure individual patient goals are achieved. Daily plans regarding ventilator management, medication titration, and other aspects of critical care must be communicated between the bedside and remote care teams to ensure individual patient goals are being met [8].

While originally conceived as a tool to improve access to intensivist-directed care, particularly in rural settings, the advantages of proactive monitoring and consistent delivery of efficacious care plans have resulted in larger centers with full-time intensivist coverage utilizing tele-ICU as a supplement to their ICU care delivery models. In this context, the motivation is often standardization of care, more uniform adherence to best practices, and leveraging a single pool of intensivist providers over a larger patient population [20]. In these institutions, tele-ICU is often utilized intermittently as adjunctive support when an in-house intensivist is called away from the ICU to evaluate new patients, perform procedures, or when simultaneously covering multiple ICUs [11]. Indeed, between 2007 and 2010, hospitals adopting tele-ICU programs were more likely to be large, urban, academic medical centers [20].

Models of Tele-ICU

As previously discussed, tele-ICU programs should be customized to meet the needs of the receiving hospital. While the individual duties and coverage time of the remote intensivist may be heterogeneous, there are generally three distinct models of tele-ICU programs.

The most common model is a hub-and-spoke organizational design (see Fig. 12.1a) [11]. In this model, the most advanced healthcare services are strategically centralized at a single center. This center or main campus is referred to as a hub. The hub is generally a larger, urban, sometimes academic facility that offers a full array of services and is home to the tele-ICU providers. The spokes represent outlying facilities that may either be owned by or contracted by affiliates of the hub. A multidisciplinary team located at the hub provides remote coverage for ICU beds at each spoke from a central location based on each spoke's individual arrangement with the hub [7]. Spokes are located within variable geographic distances from the hub [11]. The spokes offer basic levels of care that can handle the bulk of healthcare needs [22]. When the level of care for a patient exceeds the scope of practice of the spoke, the hub can be contacted through various forms of audiovisual communication to route their care toward the hub to either provide remote care or facilitate transfer to the hub.

The hub-and-spoke model has proven to be a well-designed organizational model that increases efficiency while reducing redundancy within a system [22]. By centralizing the infrequently used, specialized aspects of care, unnecessary duplication of equipment and personnel is eliminated, and cost is reduced. Additionally, the hub-and-spoke model unifies multiple healthcare facilities under one governing body, similar to central governance [22]. Protocols and policies can be developed collaboratively by expert-level clinicians at the hub to be implemented at the spokes.

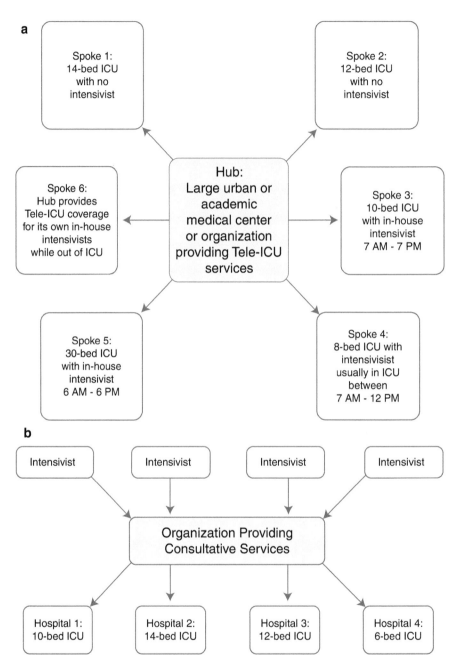

Fig. 12.1 Models of teleICU [8, 11]. (**a**) The hub-and-spoke model of ICU telehealth. The remote care team is employed by a large medical center and provides various forms of ICU coverage to regional affiliated hospitals, or spokes. (**b**) The physician service organization model is a private entity comprised of intensivist from multiple affiliations providing care to both long-distance and regional sites

This standardization of care enhances quality and delivers a consistent patient care experience across different institutions [22]. Spokes can typically be easily added on to existing hubs. Since most stand-alone hospitals do not have the resources to start their own tele-ICU program, linking to an established hub may be an attractive solution [8].

Another ICU telehealth model is the physician service organization model (Fig. 12.1b) [11]. While intensivists in a hub-and-spoke model are employed by a single flagship institution, the physician service model is comprised of individual intensivists from varying institutions and locations that form an independent, private ICU telehealth practice. In this "decentralized" model, the practice is not affiliated with any one hospital entity, and serves more as a private, "virtual" practice [7, 11]. Remote intensivists may provide coverage from their individual offices or homes supported by appropriate audiovisual technology [3, 7]. In this model, remote care is typically delivered as a specialist on-call consultative service, rather than the continuous oversight provided in the tele-ICU model [3]. This model is most similar to the use of telehealth for acute stroke care, as previously discussed. The contracting facilities in this model may be located throughout the country, or even be covered by international groups.

The third tele-ICU model is a hybrid and in this model, a physician organization group comprised of individual intensivists that form a network become affiliated with a single, tertiary care center. Although this model includes intensivists from varying institutions, it has components of a hub-and-spoke model as it focuses on centralizing care [11]. Overall, this model is less described in the literature compared to the two other models.

It is important to recognize that one model is not necessarily superior, and there is no one-size-fits all approach to tele-ICU. The inherent customizability allows tele-ICU providers to tailor their services to the needs and resources of the receiving hospital.

Tele-ICU Outcomes

Clinical Outcomes

Early tele-ICU research focused on patient mortality. The first published tele-ICU study was reported by Rosenfeld et al. [16] and showed a significant reduction in mortality and length of stay (LOS) in a community hospital surgical ICU. Since then, there have been more than 12 tele-ICU implementation studies—most using before/after study designs with adjustment for illness severity [7]. The University of Massachusetts published one of the larger scale studies of pre-and post-implementation of tele-ICU involving more than 6000 patients in 7 ICUs. The hospital mortality after implementation was 11.8% compared to 13.6% pre-implementation [23]. In addition, they noted higher adherence to best practices for preventing venous thrombosis, stress ulcers, ventilator-associated pneumonias, and catheter-related infections [23].

There have been two meta-analysis [24], one including 35 ICUs and more than 40,000 patients, showing a lower ICU mortality and length of stay with no effect on in-hospital mortality. The second meta-analysis included 11 studies [25] demonstrating lower ICU and in-hospital mortality. The included studies had a heterogeneous approach to the tele-ICU intervention and varying characterizations of program structure and implementation. A recent national study [20] to determine the effectiveness of tele-ICU used a national sample of 132 hospitals matched with 389 similar non-adopting control hospitals. They reported a small relative reduction in 90-day mortality in adopter hospitals. However, there was a wide variation in the effect across individual hospitals, with only 13% of hospitals showing a statistically significant mortality reduction after adoption. In particular, the investigators noted urban hospitals with higher case volumes derived the most benefit. Additionally, newer literature alludes to a subset of patients with higher acuity deriving more benefit from tele-ICU compared to lower acuity cohorts [2, 3].

The Critical Care Societies Collaborative—consisting of the American Association of Critical Care Nurses, American College of Chest Physicians, American Thoracic Society, and the Society of Critical Care Medicine—convened a panel to review current research conducted regarding tele-ICU [15]. The Collaborative statement concluded that key knowledge gaps include lack of granular details of ICU structure, processes of tele-ICU adoption and implementation, and inconsistency in the tele-ICU intervention approach—all confounding the scientific validity of reported clinical outcomes. Future studies will need to address these gaps with optimal control of patient, hospital, and system-level confounders.

Financial Implications

The costs associated with a tele-ICU program are a major concern for health systems, as these are not currently reimbursement by CMS or third-party payers [26]. This makes justifying the establishment of a tele-ICU program challenging, especially for resource-limited hospitals. In addition to a large initial implementation cost, there are substantial recurring costs, largely driven by personnel and licensing fees.

Initial implementation costs related to tele-ICU adoption can be variable [23]. The capabilities of the existing electronic medical record systems and technology at the receiving hospital affect the start-up and maintenance costs significantly. A functional tele-ICU program requires reliable, high-speed Internet connections to link the spoke and hub in real time. This may require hardware upgrades including more robust servers, wiring, and camera instillation. Software upgrades in electronic medical records and/or computerized physician order entry may be needed depending on what the receiving hospital already has in place. This may result in a substantial up-front investment ranging between $2 million and $5 million [27, 28].

Additionally, new training and potentially new staff in the information technology department may be needed. A report by the New England Healthcare Institute [17] provides the most detailed analysis about cost of technology, implementation, staffing fees, and operating and maintenance costs. Crude analysis by the group reports a 1-year cost ranging from $50,000 to $100,000 per ICU-bed.

Thus, tele-ICU programs typically focus substantially in financial benefits derived from the program to warrant initial and ongoing program investments. The tele-ICU return on investment is typically derived from reductions in ICU and hospital LOS, increased severity in hospital case mix index, and increase in ICU occupancy rates, and decrease in ICU transfers. Improved quality outcomes with decreased complications, mostly due to standardization of care and improved adherence to best practices, are also important determinants of the overall return on investment [3, 26, 27]. This combination of improved operational efficiency and quality of care are typically used to justify the substantial investment represented by a tele-ICU program [29].

A return on investment analysis should carefully consider particular characteristics of the hospital or health system being analyzed. For example, an analysis performed by the New England Health Care Institute on the University of Massachusetts Memorial Medical Center [17] revealed a reduction in hospital length of stay by 20% leading to an estimated 25 million dollar projected profit, but smaller hospitals with lower case volume would be unlikely to generate comparable performance. In contrast to larger, multi-ICU health systems, smaller community hospitals may derive substantial return on investment related to the ability to retain patients in their ICUs with higher acuity due to the increased support of tele-ICU [23].

A systematic review of financial implications of tele-ICU has noted a hospital profit when affiliated with a commercial vendor [27]. However, many of these studies lack precise details on breakdown of cost. Additionally, the studies propose cost savings based on surrogate ICU outcomes and indirect reimbursements but fail to provide granular data demonstrating true cost savings. While some studies have shown favorable financial gains through increased case volume, revenue, and lower cost of care [28], other studies have shown a higher cost associated with tele-ICU programs [7]. Larger, more robust studies are needed to further elucidate the cost to benefit financial performance of tele-ICU programs.

Educational Implications

Tele-ICU is becoming more prevalent in teaching hospitals with residents, fellows, and other trainees. There have been concerns of tele-ICU programs diluting the educational experience of these trainees by diluting their independence and excessive supervision by the remote intensivist. However, studies to date have not revealed these concerns to be well grounded. In fact, many trainees have welcomed the supervision and access to an extra layer of support to help reduce the emotional toll and burn out associated with caring for complex ICU patients, especially when bedside attending physicians may be absent from the ICU [1]. The remote intensivist can augment the learning of trainees by proving real-time feedback at the bedside by earlier recognition of educational gaps and opportunities. One report from a training institution where trainees rotate in medical ICUs with and without monitoring found that 82% of trainees felt tele-ICU programs improved patient care [30]. Trainees have also noted that tele-ICU providers are a valuable resource during ventilator management, code supervision, and respiratory complications. Thus, trainees perceive tele-ICU as a valuable educational experience, rather than a hindrance to learning [31]. Institutions with advanced learners, such as critical care fellows, and hospitals with night-time intensivist coverage may not experience the same educational benefits noted above.

Drivers for Tele-ICU Adoption

The need for a high performing, cost-effective critical care program is frequently the strategic driver for implementing a tele-ICU program. A strong program can favorably impact a hospital's ability to achieve the Institute of Healthcare Improvement's "Triple Aim" of improving patient care experience, improving population health, and reducing the cost of care. A robust tele-ICU, through reductions in physician on-call burden and increased nurse retention, may also improve the work-life balance of healthcare providers, which has been proposed as a fourth aim [32, 33] (Table 12.1).

ICU Physician Staffing Drivers

The Leapfrog Group [34] is a consortium of purchasers of healthcare that grades hospitals on an annual survey of quality and safety. This important consortium stipulates that to meet their standards for intensivist physician staffing, ICU patients should be managed or co-managed by a board-certified intensivist during daytime hours and this physician should not have clinical obligations external to the ICU. Additionally, when not present on site or via telemedicine, the intensivist should return alerts 95% of the time within 5 minutes and arrange for appropriate personal to reach ICU patients within 5 minutes [35]. In the Leapfrog Group's 2017 Hospital Survey, just 56% of responding hospitals met this standard [36]. Tele-ICU programs can help mitigate this quality and coverage gap through provision of 24/7 intensivist physician access, and these standards are a primary driver for the most pervasive form of tele-ICU: continuous remote monitoring.

Many acute care hospitals have no intensivist support for ICU patients. In this setting, non-critical care-trained physicians such as hospitalists provide oversight to ICU patients. A recent survey looking at the practice patterns of rural, non-intensivist hospitalists practicing in the ICU reported 66% of the hospitalists served as the

Table 12.1 The quadruple aim of drivers to teleICU adoption

Improving patient experience	Access to critical care expertise
	Adherence to best practice ICU physician staffing (e.g. Leapfrog compliance)
	Immediate physician access for patient and family
	Consistent level of care 24/7
	Improved outcomes
Improving population health	Leverage scarce intensivists
	Improved outcomes and quality of care
	Availability of acuity scored outcomes data
	Best practice compliance data for quality improvement
	Leadership support
	Improved healthcare delivery at local level
	Decreased tertiary care overload
Reducing costs of care	Cost avoidance with decreased LOS
	Improved ICU utilization and throughput
	Patient retention at community hospitals
	Improved best practice compliance
	Reduced complications
Improving healthcare provider work-life balance	Addition of critical care subspecialty expertise
	Expansion of existing critical care group
	Patient management by teleICU when on-site physician involved with other responsibilities
	ICU leadership support
	Nursing support for patient management

ICU intensive care unit, *LOS* length of stay

primary physicians in the ICU, and 50% felt obliged to practice beyond their scope of practice [37]. This reveals that these physicians, lacking intensivist support, are frequently uncomfortable and not adequately trained to manage critically ill patients [37].

For hospitals with some access to intensivist-directed care, the tele-ICU creates an effectively larger critical care practice group. This enables the bedside intensivists to have more flexibility and broader reach in meeting their multiple responsibilities. Indeed, in this practice context hospital administration concerns about burnout in their bedside physician staff is a strong influencer in the decision to implement a tele-ICU program [11, 27]. With regard to acceptability of tele-ICU programs among ICU staff, evaluations of staff acceptance of tele-ICU have shown high rates of satisfaction after implementation of tele-ICU due to improved perception of patient care, communication, reduced workload, and enhanced hospital reputation [3, 21, 38]. The mechanism for improved satisfaction may be derived from providing staff with rapid access to an intensivist when bedside physicians have competing obligations [3, 11].

While larger academic institutions are more likely to have 24/7 bedside intensivists, such organizations are often challenged by high patient volumes and related capacity strain. It has been demonstrated in an academic institution that a single intensivist should only concurrently manage up to 14 patients; however, this ratio is often exceeded [39]. The tele-ICU intensivist, on the other hand, can cover approximately 10–15 times the volume of patients. Thus, the tele-ICU model could supplement the bedside intensivist and may expand their coverage capabilities.

Quality of ICU Care Drivers

The desire to improve quality in the existing ICU operations is another key driver for tele-ICU adoption. Operational data made available for public review through efforts such as Leapfrog and CMS quality initiatives and an increasing number of best practices and practice guidelines have prompted hospital leaders to recognize the need to standardize care within individual hospitals and across their health systems. This standardization requires leadership, ICU-specific data, and a consistent approach to compliance at all times of the day/night/weekend.

The dedication of an institution to develop a robust quality improvement program may influence the decision to implement the continuous tele-ICU model. The availability of severity-of-illness adjusted outcomes data and evidence-based practice compliance that can be collected by the tele-ICU data collection team is an important institutional quality improvement tool and allows hospitals to benchmark their performance against local and national standards [7]. Tele-ICU programs can generate reports regarding adherence to best practice guidelines, which simultaneously improve patient outcomes and reduce cost [1, 7]. In many ways, this may be the most efficacious feature of tele-ICU. The ability to consistently implement high-quality, evidenced-based care may have a greater role in improved patient outcomes and reduced ICU and hospital expenses more than the ability to provide continuous physiologic monitoring [3, 7].

In community hospitals, ICU medical directors have numerous competing responsibilities [40] and are frequently limited in their availability and ability to implement current evidence-based best practices. Many community hospitals engage with and utilize a tele-ICU to provide leadership support and ICU performance data to drive improvements in quality of care. Prolonged ICU LOS and ventilator days are a frequent focus for quality improvement. A highly involved tele-ICU can provide tools and staff to impact both [23, 41]. This is reflected in the published decrease in mortality and improved compliance with best practices reviewed earlier.

Financial Drivers

There is a financial cost to an institution for ICUs with underperforming quality of care. This is reflected in prolonged length of stay, poor outcomes, safety events, and potential lawsuits. ICU costs can run as high as 20–30% of total hospital costs [42,

43]. Decreasing LOS benefits the hospital financially through decreased variable cost and availability of additional beds for new patient admissions. In addition to impacting LOS, an effective tele-ICU program applies the data collected to optimize ICU bed utilization and throughput so that patients are admitted to an appropriate, and safe level of care.

Patient retention as a result of availability of critical care expertise can add direct revenue to the hospital. Analogous to the University of Massachusetts' experience, in the author's experience of over 15 years in tele-ICU, community hospitals have been able to retain patients they were previously transferring, particularly in hospitals with limited critical care/intensivist subspecialty support. Related to patient retention and growth, the availability of intensivists who can manage sicker patients is an important calculation when hospitals decide to implement a new service line such as cardiac catheterization with percutaneous coronary intervention or cardiovascular surgery. A tele-ICU program can support these growth initiatives. Patient retention in community hospitals has a broader impact on controlling healthcare costs. Managing common critical illnesses in community hospitals has been shown to be more cost-effective than transferring them to a tertiary center [17]. This also relieves congestion at the tertiary centers, opening beds for patients requiring services that are only available at those centers. Keeping patients in their own communities can also improve patient and family satisfaction with local hospitals [11].

The decision to build a tele-ICU or collaborate with or contract the service from an existing tele-ICU vendor depends on the size and availability of staff to provide the service as well as an analysis of the costs to build and support the program. As previously mentioned, community hospitals may be best served by obtaining tele-ICU services from an existing tele-ICU provider due to the financial and staffing barriers of creating their own system de novo. Larger hospital systems and academic medical centers may have the options of building their own tele-ICU program, collaborating with an existing tele-ICU provider, or purchasing the service from a third-party tele-ICU vendor.

Barriers to Tele-ICU Implementation

Once a hospital or hospital system decides pursuing a tele-ICU program is a priority, there are some common barriers and challenges that need to be addressed. Table 12.2 highlights the more commonly encountered barriers and strategies to overcome the resistance to implementation [1, 6, 21, 44].

Drivers of Success and Sustainability

Although a growing body of research has evaluated telehealth's clinical and financial value in hospitals' ICUs, most studies have used "before-and-after" designs, typically single center, to measure the impact of ICU telehealth on conventional

Table 12.2 Barriers to implementing teleICU programs and strategies to overcome these obstacles

Category	Barrier	Strategy to overcome
Physician	Fear of negative financial impact on their consultative practice Replacement by teleICU program Loss of autonomy	Education regarding goals and limits of the teleICU Reinforcing teleICU as a support system Clearly defining teleICU responsibilities and autonomy Regular in-person meetings between teleICU and local physicians
Cost and reimbursement	Larger initial cost: investment in hardware and systems upgrades, operations center space Physician licensing costs (if covering other states) Maintaining software, upgrades Information technology (IT) department costs Reimbursement is limited/non-existant and varies between states Providers cannot charge critical care professional fees for teleICU	Leverage cost against indirect savings to hospitals Apply for external funding (e.g. grants) Utilize established teleICU vendors to offset some of the initial cost as opposed to starting de novo
ICU staffing	Collaboration with another service and additional hand-offs Increased workloads will lead to burnout and attrition Poor provider buy-in	Designate ICU champions to demonstrate feasibility and improved care Make teleICU provider part of already-occurring handoffs Periodic site visits to increase rapport and host feedback sessions
Information technology	Hardware instillation cost—computer monitors, possible internet server upgrades Software development and upgrades Time and availability to troubleshoot Staff education on how to use technology	Designate champions to become experts with the technology to reach other staff members Possible collaboration between provider and site IT departments Utilize established third-party providers
Licensure and credentialing	Tele-ICU providers must be licensed in each state they practice Tele-ICU providers are members of medical staff at each hospital they provide coverage for, and are subject to each individual hospital's rules, regulations, and policies	TeleICU vendors can hire a credentialing expert to keep licensures and privileges updated
Legal and regulatory aspects	All equipment must be HIPAA compliant Tele-ICU providers are responsible and liable for medical decisions they make	Because providers may be entering their own orders, directly interacting with patient/staff, viewing trends, and documenting their patient interventions, overall there is reduced me dico-legal risk

Table 12.3 Factors that affect success and sustainability

Organizational factors	Site-specific structural, cultural, or human factors impacting how much benefit a site derives from ICU telehealth (e.g., critical care committee structure, physician leadership, staff buy-in)
Clinical factors	ICU telehealth's ability to drive improvements in clinical quality metrics (e.g., ICU mortality, readmissions, protocol adherence rates)
Financial factors	ICU telehealth's ability to drive revenue growth and/or cost reduction (e.g., ICU volume, length-of-stay, bed utilization)
Strategic factors	ICU telehealth's impact on clinical staff satisfaction, organizational reputation, and organizational plans for future resource deployment (e.g., physician retention, patient satisfaction, physician recruitment)

outcomes measures (e.g., ICU mortality and length of stay) [24, 25, 27, 45, 46]. While this method can offer insight into specific aspects of hospital and ICU performance, it lacks broader strategic perspective and is prone to scientific weaknesses and lack of practical applicability [47, 48]. Furthermore, from a clinical program perspective, there is substantial variation in the organizational specifics (e.g., staffing, hours of operation, data reporting) of different tele-ICU programs making it difficult to compare results [48–50]. Additionally, hospitals that have already adopted tele-ICU currently lack a strategic framework through which they can efficiently analyze and improve their performance. Table 12.3 highlights factors that could be taken into account to measure success and sustainability of a tele-ICU program [51].

Future Directions

Tele-ICU has evolved substantially since its first introduction more than 20 years ago. The shortage of intensivists and capacity strain at tertiary facilities appear to make ongoing expansion of a leveraged model of critical care inevitable. Additionally, as reimbursement migrates from a fee-for-service structure toward emphasis on payments linked to quality and outcomes, as well as bundled payments, managing the quality and costs of critical care will become increasingly important to acute care hospitals. As technology continues to evolve and data acquisition and application grow in importance, tele-ICU programs will also need to evolve. Short-term areas ripe for development should include smart decision support and artificial intelligence tools capable of analyzing and simplifying the vast quantity of patient data into meaningful, actionable information while minimizing artifact.

In this rapidly evolving area, there needs to be a balance between premature investment in unproven technology-based service industries and waiting too long for lengthy trials to prove efficacy. Ultimately, the clinical, financial, and personnel impacts of tele-ICU programs will drive continued growth [15]. Each hospital system and individual hospital will need to evaluate what combination of on-site and telehealth support will best help achieve the quadruple aim of healthcare.

References

1. Lilly CM, Zubrow MT, Kempner KM, Reynolds HN, Subramanian S, Eriksson EA, et al. Critical care telemedicine: evolution and state of the art. Crit Care Med. 2014;42(11):2429–36.
2. Udeh C, Udeh B, Rahman N, Canfield C, Campbell J, Hata JS. Telemedicine/virtual ICU: where are we and where are we going? Methodist Debakey Cardiovasc J. 2018;14(2):126–33.
3. Fuhrman SA, Lilly CM. ICU telemedicine solutions. Clin Chest Med. 2015;36(3):401–7.
4. EM D. The critical care workforce. Senate Report. 2013:109–43.
5. Zawada ET Jr, Herr P, Larson D, Fromm R, Kapaska D, Erickson D. Impact of an intensive care unit telemedicine program on a rural health care system. Postgrad Med. 2009;121(3):160–70.
6. Kahn JM, Rak KJ, Kuza CC, Ashcraft LE, Barnato AE, Fleck JC, et al. Determinants of intensive care unit telemedicine effectiveness: an ethnographic study. Am J Respir Crit Care Med. 2018;199:970.
7. Vranas KC, Slatore CG, Kerlin MP. Telemedicine coverage of intensive care units: a narrative review. Ann Am Thorac Soc. 2018;15:1256.
8. Breslow MJ. Remote ICU care programs: current status. J Crit Care. 2007;22(1):66–76.
9. Lilly CM, McLaughlin JM, Zhao H, Baker SP, Cody S, Irwin RS, et al. A multicenter study of ICU telemedicine reengineering of adult critical care. Chest. 2014;145(3):500–7.
10. Becker C, Frishman WH, Scurlock C. Telemedicine and teleICU: the evolution and differentiation of a new medical field. Am J Med. 2016;129(12):e333–e4.
11. Rogove H. How to develop a teleICU model? Crit Care Nurs Q. 2012;35(4):357–63.
12. Demaerschalk BM, Miley ML, Kiernan TE, Bobrow BJ, Corday DA, Wellik KE, et al. Stroke telemedicine. Mayo Clin Proc. 2009;84(1):53–64.
13. Wechsler LR. Advantages and limitations of teleneurology. JAMA Neurol. 2015;72(3):349–54.
14. Al Kasab S, Adams RJ, Debenham E, Jones DJ, Holmstedt CA. Medical University of South Carolina Telestroke: a telemedicine facilitated network for stroke treatment in South Carolina-a progress report. Telemed J E Health. 2017;23(8):674–7.
15. Kahn JM, Hill NS, Lilly CM, Angus DC, Jacobi J, Rubenfeld GD, et al. The research agenda in ICU telemedicine: a statement from the Critical Care Societies Collaborative. Chest. 2011;140(1):230–8.
16. Rosenfeld BA, Dorman T, Breslow MJ, Pronovost P, Jenckes M, Zhang N, et al. Intensive care unit telemedicine: alternate paradigm for providing continuous intensivist care. Crit Care Med. 2000;28(12):3925–31.
17. Collaborative NEHIaMI. The case for Tele-ICU in Intensive Care. USA 2010.
18. Sapirstein A, Lone N, Latif A, Fackler J, Pronovost PJ. Tele ICU: paradox or panacea? Best Pract Res Clin Anaesthesiol. 2009;23(1):115–26.
19. Lilly CM, Thomas EJ. Tele-ICU: experience to date. J Intensive Care Med. 2010;25(1):16–22.
20. Kahn JM, Cicero BD, Wallace DJ, Iwashyna TJ. Adoption of ICU telemedicine in the United States. Crit Care Med. 2014;42(2):362–8.
21. Kumar S, Merchant S, Reynolds R. Tele-ICU: efficacy and cost-effectiveness of remotely managing critical care. Perspect Health Inf Manag. 2013;1f:10.
22. Elrod JK, Fortenberry JL Jr. The hub-and-spoke organization design: an avenue for serving patients well. BMC Health Serv Res. 2017;17(Suppl 1):457.
23. Lilly CM, Cody S, Zhao H, Landry K, Baker SP, McIlwaine J, et al. Hospital mortality, length of stay, and preventable complications among critically ill patients before and after teleICU reengineering of critical care processes. JAMA. 2011;305(21):2175–83.
24. Young LB, Chan PS, Lu X, Nallamothu BK, Sasson C, Cram PM. Impact of telemedicine intensive care unit coverage on patient outcomes: a systematic review and meta-analysis. Arch Intern Med. 2011;171(6):498–506.
25. Wilcox ME, Adhikari NK. The effect of telemedicine in critically ill patients: systematic review and meta-analysis. Crit Care. 2012;16(4):R127.
26. Kruklitis RJ, Tracy JA, McCambridge MM. Clinical and financial considerations for implementing an ICU telemedicine program. Chest. 2014;145(6):1392–6.

27. Kumar G, Falk DM, Bonello RS, Kahn JM, Perencevich E, Cram P. The costs of critical care telemedicine programs: a systematic review and analysis. Chest. 2013;143(1):19–29.
28. Breslow MJ, Rosenfeld BA, Doerfler M, Burke G, Yates G, Stone DJ, et al. Effect of a multiple-site intensive care unit telemedicine program on clinical and economic outcomes: an alternative paradigm for intensivist staffing. Crit Care Med. 2004;32(1):31–8.
29. Lilly CM, Motzkus C, Rincon T, Cody SE, Landry K, Irwin RS, et al. ICU Telemedicine Program Financial Outcomes. Chest. 2017;151(2):286–97.
30. Kuszler PC. Telemedicine and integrated health care delivery: compounding malpractice liability. Am J Law Med. 1999;25(2–3):297–326.
31. Coletti C, Elliott DJ, Zubrow MT. Resident perceptions of a tele-intensive care unit implementation. Telemed J E Health. 2010;16(8):894–7.
32. Bodenheimer T, Sinsky C. From triple to quadruple aim: care of the patient requires care of the provider. Ann Fam Med. 2014;12(6):573–6.
33. Anandarajah AP, Quill TE, Privitera MR. Adopting the quadruple aim: the University of Rochester Medical Center experience: moving from physician burnout to physician resilience. Am J Med. 2018;131:979.
34. Group CHaTL. ICU physician staffing. 2016.; Available from: http://www.leapfroggroup.org/sites/default/files/Files/Castlight-Leapfrog-ICU-Physician-Staffing-Report-2016.pdf.
35. Leapfrog Hospital Survey. Factsheet: ICU physician staffing. [updated 4/1/2019Accessed March 29, 2019]; Available from: http://www.leapfroggroup.org/sites/default/files/Files/2019%20IPS%20Fact%20Sheet.pdf.
36. Angus DC, Shorr AF, White A, Dremsizov TT, Schmitz RJ, Kelley MA, et al. Critical care delivery in the United States: distribution of services and compliance with Leapfrog recommendations. Crit Care Med. 2006;34(4):1016–24.
37. Sweigart JR, Aymond D, Burger A, Kelly A, Marzano N, McIlraith T, et al. Characterizing hospitalist practice and perceptions of critical care delivery. J Hosp Med. 2018;13(1):6–12.
38. Young LB, Chan PS, Cram P. Staff acceptance of teleICU coverage: a systematic review. Chest. 2011;139(2):279–88.
39. Ward NS, Afessa B, Kleinpell R, Tisherman S, Ries M, Howell M, et al. Intensivist/patient ratios in closed ICUs: a statement from the Society of Critical Care Medicine taskforce on ICU staffing. Crit Care Med. 2013;41(2):638–45.
40. Groeger JS, Strosberg MA, Halpern NA, Raphaely RC, Kaye WE, Guntupalli KK, et al. Descriptive analysis of critical care units in the United States. Crit Care Med. 1992;20(6):846–63.
41. Kalb T, Raikhelkar J, Meyer S, Ntimba F, Thuli J, Gorman MJ, et al. A multicenter population-based effectiveness study of teleintensive care unit-directed ventilator rounds demonstrating improved adherence to a protective lung strategy, decreased ventilator duration, and decreased intensive care unit mortality. J Crit Care. 2014;29(4):691 e7-14.
42. Guidet BV, Andreas, Flaatan H. Quality management in the intensive care. Cambidge, UK: Cambidge University Press; 2016.
43. Norris C, Jacobs P, Rapoport J, Hamilton S. ICU and non-ICU cost per day. Can J Anaesth. 1995;42(3):192–6.
44. Thomas EJ, Lucke JF, Wueste L, Weavind L, Patel B. Association of telemedicine for remote monitoring of intensive care patients with mortality, complications, and length of stay. JAMA. 2009;302(24):2671–8.
45. Kahn JM, Le TQ, Barnato AE, Hravnak M, Kuza CC, Pike F, et al. ICU telemedicine and critical care mortality: a National Effectiveness Study. Med Care. 2016;54(3):319–25.
46. Chen J, Sun D, Yang W, Liu M, Zhang S, Peng J, et al. Clinical and economic outcomes of telemedicine programs in the intensive care unit: a systematic review and meta-analysis. J Intensive Care Med. 2018;33(7):383–93.
47. Kahn JM, Hill NS, Lilly CM, Angus DC, Jacobi J, Rubenfeld GD, et al. The research agenda in ICU telemedicine: a statement from the critical care societies collaborative. Chest. 2011;140(1):230–8.
48. Kahn JM. ICU telemedicine: from theory to practice. Crit Care Med. 2014;42(11):2457–8.

49. Trombley MJ, Hassol A, Lloyd JT, Buchman TG, Marier AF, White A, et al. The impact of enhanced critical care training and 24/7 (teleICU) support on medicare spending and postdischarge utilization patterns. Health Serv Res. 2017;53:2099.
50. Buchman TG, Coopersmith CM, Meissen HW, Grabenkort WR, Bakshi V, Hiddleson CA, et al. Innovative interdisciplinary strategies to address the intensivist shortage. Crit Care Med. 2017;45(2):298–304.
51. Nadig NRHL, Slenzak D, McElligott J, Valenta S, Warr E, Beeks R, Ford DW. Value scorecard as teleICU evaluation tool. San Deigo: American Thoracic Society; 2018.

Index